Praise for *Bodies on the Line*

"*Bodies on the Line* tells the stories of communities that came together . . . to offer patients comfort and protection . . . The book comes at a critical moment for the constitutional right to abortion in the United States . . . The very need for clinic escort teams is a testament to the inability of current laws to secure safe, comfortable care for patients."   —*The New York Times Book Review*

"In [*Bodies on the Line*], Rankin, a writer and expert on abortion rights, traces the history of clinic escorts and defenders in the U.S. from the earliest days of legalized abortion in the 1970s through the present day . . . Rankin's research for the book is methodical and exhaustive. By not engaging in discursive debates and wild speculation on politics and legislation, Rankin keeps the book focused on the human-level experience of escorts and patients."
—Carlie Willsie, *Ms.*

"Rankin's passion for women's health blazes on the page, and she is adept at connecting disparate events to create a cohesive historical narrative . . . A stunning, compassionate history of an overlooked element within the abortion-rights movement in the U.S."
—*Kirkus Reviews* (starred review)

"A powerful tribute to abortion clinic escorts . . . Lucidly written and sharply argued, this is a sobering and timely dispatch from the fight to preserve abortion rights."   —*Publishers Weekly* (starred review)

"A must-read to understand the physical and emotional labor that comes with the fight to ensure that abortion is both accessible and a human right."   —*Electric Literature*

"This history of abortion clinic escorts in the United States by writer and activist Rankin is timely, engaging, and full of compassion . . . This sweeping history will leave readers wanting to learn more. It is both a celebration of devoted volunteer clinic escorts and a call to action to improve the circumstances under which people seek health care." —*Library Journal*

"*Bodies on the Line* tells the story of the unsung heroes who have done so much to help women exercise their reproductive rights—clinic escorts. Who they are, why they're there, and what they have endured is mind-boggling, frustrating, and ultimately inspiring. Americans owe a debt to these volunteer activists who literally put their bodies on the line for those rights"
—Elisa Camahort Page, coauthor of *Road Map for Revolutionaries: Resistance, Activism, and Advocacy for All*

"Where the law has failed to protect abortion patients, grassroots activists have kept showing up. *Bodies on the Line* is an impressively reported, compassionate chronicle of what it means to truly support abortion access, and the story it tells couldn't be more timely."
—Irin Carmon, coauthor of the *New York Times* bestseller *Notorious RBG*

"*Bodies on the Line* edified me and enraged me—and it also gave me hope." —Moira Donegan, columnist at *The Guardian*

"*Bodies on the Line* is a story of the courage, hope, and defiance embodied by generations of clinic escorts and activists—and a timely reminder that the fight for safe and legal abortion has always unfolded not only in courtrooms and legislatures, but in our communities.

With this book, Lauren Rankin urges readers to be part of shaping the future of reproductive rights in America."

—Cecile Richards, former president of Planned Parenthood and *New York Times* bestselling author of *Make Trouble*

"I have long admired Lauren's work and am thrilled to learn that she's writing a book about one of the most undercovered and crucial, life-saving, rigorous forms of activism out there . . . Brings me hope and joy in a period in which those two things can be sorely lacking."

—Rebecca Traister, *New York Times* bestselling author of *All the Single Ladies*

"*Bodies on the Line* is an exciting history of clinic escorting. The people who do this work have helped shape access to abortion in America. While I wish this work and such a book were not needed, everyone needs to know this story and why it matters."

—Dr. Jen Gunter, *New York Times* bestselling author of *The Vagina Bible*

"Lauren Rankin's passionate defense of women's reproductive rights is inspiring. She is on the forefront of this incredibly important issue."

—Shannon Watts, founder of Moms Demand Action for Gun Sense in America

"Lauren Rankin has written a testament to the humanity that is central to the procedure, and the act, of abortion. She has walked the walk, and shared with other dedicated clinic escorts the fear and the dehumanization, and the threats, that patients face every time they walk into a clinic to receive basic health care. Here, directly from the front lines, are unique and untold stories that broaden our understanding of what it takes today for people to get the care they deserve, what we stand to lose when they can't, and what we need to do if we're to see our right to bodily autonomy fully realized. *Bodies on the Line* is an essential read for this moment of crisis."

—Martha Plimpton, actor, activist, and cofounder of A is For

BODIES on the LINE

BODIES on the LINE

At the Front Lines of the Fight

to Protect Abortion in America

LAUREN RANKIN

COUNTERPOINT
BERKELEY, CALIFORNIA

The Library of Congress has cataloged the hardcover edition as follows:
Names: Rankin, Lauren, author.
Title: Bodies on the line : at the front lines of the fight to protect
abortion in America / Lauren Rankin.
Description: First hardcover edition. | Berkeley, California :
Counterpoint, 2022. | Includes bibliographical references.
Identifiers: LCCN 2021037793 | ISBN 9781640094741 (hardcover) |
ISBN 9781640094758 (ebook)
Subjects: LCSH: Abortion—United States. | Health services
accessibility—United States. | Abortion services—United States—
Employees | Pro-choice movement—United States.
Classification: LCC HQ767.5.U5 R36 2022 | DDC 362.1988/800973—dc23
LC record available at https://lccn.loc.gov/2021037793

Paperback ISBN: 978-1-64009-591-5

Cover design by Dana Li
Book design by Wah-Ming Chang

COUNTERPOINT
2560 Ninth Street, Suite 318
Berkeley, CA 94710
www.counterpointpress.com

Printed in the United States of America
1 3 5 7 9 10 8 6 4 2

For Drew and Elodie

I stand up, and this one of me
turns into a hundred of me.
They say I circle around you.
Nonsense. I circle around me.

—Rumi

Contents

CONTENTS

Preface

So That Happened

WHEN *BODIES ON THE LINE* WAS FIRST RELEASED IN HARD-cover in April 2022, the landscape for abortion rights in the United States already looked bleak. Texas had enacted SB8, which banned abortions at six weeks and deputized private citizens to sue to enforce it. The Supreme Court heard oral arguments in *Dobbs v. Jackson Women's Health Organization*, centered on the constitutionality of Mississippi's fifteen-week abortion ban. It was a direct challenge to *Roe v. Wade*, and the conservative justices on the Supreme Court sounded hostile to that precedent. I knew that some of the clinics that I featured in this book were in danger of being forced to close, that some abortion bans would ultimately be allowed to go into effect.

Less than a month after my book came out, a leaked draft of the Supreme Court's opinion in *Dobbs* landed like the bombshell it was—the Court was going to overturn *Roe v. Wade* and *Planned Parenthood v. Casey*, ending the constitutional right to an abortion. It wasn't official yet, but there it was, in black and white: the end of *Roe v. Wade*.

Just a few weeks after its release, my book was "timely," coming "at a critical moment." A few interviewers even asked me if I had planned this. I would awkwardly laugh. "No," I'd say. "I didn't plan for any of this."

I had long suspected, however, that *Roe v. Wade*'s days were numbered. Amy Coney Barrett's appointment to the Supreme Court in October 2020 felt like the beginning of the end for *Roe*—now the conservatives didn't even need Chief Justice John Roberts's vote to end *Roe*. During the December 2021 oral arguments in *Dobbs v. Jackson Women's Health Organization*, the conservative justices openly signaled their hostility to *Roe* and their willingness to end it. And that's just what they did on the morning of June 24, 2022.

The final ruling in *Dobbs* was essentially the same as the leaked draft. *Roe v. Wade* and *Planned Parenthood v. Casey* were overruled, and abortion's legality was now kicked back to the states. Within a matter of days, abortion was banned in Missouri, Oklahoma, and Texas, and the ban kept spreading. Horrific news stories of ten-year-old rape victims being forced to travel out of state for an abortion became our new normal. Concern that emergency contraception and long-acting reversible contraceptives like IUDs could become illegal took hold. A wave of newly registered female voters caused speculation on how this issue would affect the midterm elections. After decades of trying to ignore it, suddenly the issue of abortion was *everywhere*.

In the aftermath of *Roe*'s end, we have once again ended up where we started—abortion is a political football. We hear the latest on which states have abortion bans in effect. But what about the human impact of those bans? What about the toll it takes for a pregnant person to not only decide to have an abortion, but figure out a way to travel hundreds, even thousands, of miles away just to get one? What about the staff at clinics across the South and Midwest who are now unemployed because the kind of health-care provision they specialized in is now a crime? What about the college-bound teenagers who are now afraid of what might happen when they go away to school in a state where abortion is banned? Or the pregnant cancer patient who can't access the treatment they need to survive because it could negatively affect their fetus?

I know it feels dire right now. The consequences of the end of *Roe v. Wade*, which we've only begun to see, are already horrifying enough, and it will likely get worse. Since *Roe* fell, total or near-total abortion bans have gone into effect in fourteen states. Of the clinics in those states, nearly two-thirds have been forced to stop providing abortion care, and a third of them have closed completely.[1] Several of the clinics that I feature in this book are now indeed closed: Jackson Women's Health Organization (or the Pinkhouse, as it was commonly known) in Mississippi, the Houston Women's Clinic in Texas, EMW Women's Surgical Center in Kentucky, Whole Woman's Health in Fort Worth, Texas, and more. Others, like Red River Women's Clinic in North Dakota, were forced to move to another state to continue providing abortion care. The landscape is rapidly shifting, and what's true today might not be true tomorrow.

But what remains true is the spirit of this book and the incredible clinic escorts, staff, and patients I feature within it. It is an undeniable national tragedy that *Roe v. Wade* was overturned, yes, but abortion access was crippled long before *Roe* finally died. And yet the people in this book refused to allow abortion restrictions, mass protests, and acts of violence to deter them from showing up to protect abortion patients and ensure that they could still get this care. Time and again, they have put their bodies on the line for the rights of others, and they've done it without seeking attention or praise. That spirit is needed, now more than ever, as we enter the undoubtedly dark days to come.

Roe v. Wade doesn't exist anymore, but that doesn't mean that the fight for access to safe abortion care is over. Let the lessons of our forebearers edify and inspire you. There is work to be done. Here's to those who, even in the despondency of this moment, continue to do it.

BODIES on the LINE

Introduction

How Did We Get Here?

"You cannot block the car," I told the bodies amassed in front of the cab. "That is against the law!"

"We don't have to listen to you!" a man yelled back as he elbowed past me. "You're not better than us!"

By that bright August morning in 2015, it had been more than a year and a half since I began volunteering as a clinic escort at Metropolitan Medical Associates clinic in northern New Jersey. I had no idea what a clinic escort was when I started, much less why it was necessary. I didn't really know that abortion clinics still experienced aggression and hostility, that dozens of picketers showed up on any given day to yell at anyone who walked into a clinic. And I certainly didn't understand how important clinic escorts were in supporting patients and making abortion access a reality. I would quickly learn.

I turned my attention back to the cab. This Saturday morning started like most—a handful of agitators buzzing around—but by the time that cab pulled up, dozens of angry protesters had filled the sidewalk outside the clinic, and they were amped up. Now they had completely blocked the rear doors of the cab, shoving their signs into the windows and screaming at the people sitting in the back seat. It was impossible for anyone to get in or out of that cab.

I felt anger rising in my gut, panic building in my toes. I wanted to scream at them, push them out of the way. But I couldn't. I knew that wouldn't help. *Stay calm,* I told myself. *You can't afford to lose control. Just find a way to get to that back seat.*

My bright yellow vest, with the words CLINIC ESCORT VOLUNTEER printed across the chest, did absolutely nothing to encourage this mass of antiabortion protesters to clear the way for whoever was seated in the back. It was my job to get to them, to help them out of the car, to support them and walk them past this hostile group. I was a clinic escort. I was supposed to be their lifeline, their support. I put my body on the line for theirs.

But in that moment, there was no way for me to get to the cab without physically moving bodies, and I wasn't allowed to do that. My clinic escort team practiced strict nonengagement, which meant that we couldn't even speak to the protesters, let alone touch them. Even if they elbowed or shoved one of us (and they certainly did), we couldn't reciprocate. There was only one thing left for me to do. I held the walkie-talkie close to my lips. "Security, I need you," I said. "*Now.*"

As the security guard barreled through the front door toward us, I glanced from left to right, trying to keep tabs on the additional protesters that orbited the mob. "I doubt anyone wants to go to jail today," the guard muttered. Just like that, the mob dispersed, parting like the Red Sea. He poked his head in the back seat, beckoning whoever was in there to come on out. Another clinic escort and I were beside him. As soon as the woman emerged, I wrapped my arm around her. I pivoted my body, a stranger tucked into my left side, and used my right arm to create a barrier between her and the protesters, who were desperately trying to get in her face. I took a step and so did she, in tandem, one after the other.

It was just the two of us, together, in that moment. The mass of bodies through which I navigated our two bodies, the cacophony around us—"Don't murder your baby!" "*No mate a su hijo!*" "You'll still be the mother, just the mother of a dead baby!"—faded into the background as I narrowed my focus to a singular goal: get her in the door.

"It's all going to be okay," I said in a low, soothing tone. "Keep listening to my voice. The door is right over there. We're so close, just stay with me and stay with my voice. Everything is going to be all right."

It took the blink of an eye, or a lifetime, to reach that door.

The door closed behind us, and we were suddenly enveloped in silence. I finally looked—really looked—at who I had just escorted. Her baby face was frozen in fear, her hands clenched in tiny, defensive fists. This wasn't a woman at all. This was just a girl, and she was absolutely terrified.

"It's over now," I said. "You're inside. You're safe."

She collapsed into me, heaving, releasing guttural sobs into my chest. I held her, slowly rocking her back and forth. The security guard moved back behind the plexiglass barrier to his seat.

"It's okay," I repeated. "It's all going to be okay. You're inside. They can't get you in here. You're safe. It's okay."

We rocked, back and forth, back and forth, for another minute. Or another hour.

The front door opened. Another woman shuffled in, flanked by my fellow clinic escort. The girl in my arms looked up, recognizing her mother, and started sobbing again. Her mother held her, checked her in to the clinic, and walked into the waiting room. She was in. She was going to be okay.

I took a breath, gently chewing the side of my cheek as the adrenaline started to wane.

"You okay?" the security guard asked.

"Yeah, I'm fine." I wasn't, really, but I didn't have any other choice. There were more patients coming, more people to walk through the gauntlet. I opened the clinic's front door, slamming it against the outer brick wall. I stared at the group of protesters, meeting their hostile gaze with an inner fire that, until that moment, I didn't know I had.

"I'm calling the cops on the next person to try something like that," I wanted to scream at them. I wanted to tell them how cruel they were, how despicable their behavior was, how furious it made me to see what they did to that young girl whose tears now stained my vest.

Instead, I walked over to the next car. It started anew.

• • •

On May 17, 2021, the Supreme Court announced that it would hear oral arguments in *Dobbs v. Jackson Women's Health*, a challenge to Mississippi's ban on abortions at fifteen weeks.[1] A year later, on June 24, 2022, the ruling in that case became official: the Supreme Court overturned *Roe v. Wade*, ending the constitutional right to abortion in the United States.

Today, most people of reproductive age in the United States were born post-*Roe* (myself included), in a world where legal abortion was a given. That right had already been fought for and won, we were raised to think. If you ever needed an abortion, you could just go to a clinic and get one, right?

Now, half a century later, we are left to reckon with what once seemed so unthinkable. How did we get here? How did abortion become illegal across vast swaths of the country? How did we end up in a post-*Roe* America?

It has happened slowly, under our noses, for decades. For just as long as there has been legal abortion in the United States, there has been a dedicated and concerted effort to undermine it. The crisis point at which *Roe v. Wade* now finds itself is the result of years of restrictions and bans, yes, but also a coordinated effort to if not outright ban abortion, then make it as difficult to get as humanly possible.

Nowhere is that clearer than outside the front door of an abortion clinic.

If you live in one of the 10 percent of U.S. counties that still has an abortion clinic, there is probably a group of picketers outside of it right now.[2] They might be holding gruesome signs with doctored photos of bloody fetuses. Some might be yelling into megaphones, accosting every person who walks by the clinic. Others are probably holding up their cell phones, capturing patients' faces as they enter the clinic's doors, posting them online when they get home. They're swarming patients' cars. Then they're slamming their signs into car windows. And they're shouting, "Don't murder your baby!" in a girl's face. For blocks, they follow people. "You're going to hell," they shout. "You're going to die inside that butcher shop!" They pray and prey, over and over again.

Their goal? To make it as difficult and traumatic as possible to access an abortion.

Abortion opponents have admitted as much. In a 2018 NPR interview with Terry Gross, Reverend Robert Schenck, a former militant antiabortion protester in the 1980s and '90s, explained their rationale and tactics: "Of course we engaged in mass blockades. Sometimes we would have a dozen people in front of the doorways to a clinic. Other times, it would be hundreds. On occasion, we actually had thousands. We created human obstacles for those coming and going, whether they were the abortion providers themselves, their staff members, of course women and sometimes men accompanying them that would come to the clinics. And it created a very intimidating encounter."[3]

That balmy August morning that I held a sobbing teenager in my arms wasn't an anomaly but a regular occurrence. Actually stopping someone from having an abortion isn't protesters' *entire* goal—they want to stigmatize abortion, to force everyone who ends up choosing to have one to experience personal suffering because of it.

"I remember women—some of them quite young—being very distraught," Reverend Schenck repentantly told Terry Gross. "Over time, I became very callous to that. They were more objects than they were human beings with real feelings in real personal crisis."[4]

For nearly as long as abortion clinics have been open for business in this country, there have been violent opponents outside their front doors. They came in droves to shut down abortion clinics with their voices and their bodies.

Local police didn't stop them. Neither did presidents, or even the Supreme Court. What ultimately held the increasingly chaotic protesters at bay wasn't the law—it was volunteers. It was clinic escorts.

Beginning in the late 1970s, in response to the growing virulence outside abortion clinics across the country, ragtag groups of activists came together to do something about it: walk the patients inside. It sounds absurd in its simplicity—just walk with people—but that's what makes it so radical.

For many abortion patients, from the moment they exit their car until the moment the clinic doors close behind them, they are bombarded by dozens, hundreds, even thousands of people yelling at them, telling them to turn around, handing them literature filled with junk science, shoving cameras into their faces. The dehumanization that Reverend Schenck described wasn't an accident, but the very point. Even seeing one warm face, having one supportive body next to them, can help put a patient at ease, or at the very least help them follow through on the choice they've already made for themselves.

Clinic escorts have played a vital role in facilitating abortion access since the very beginning of legal abortion in the United States. These volunteers, and the organizers who helped corral them into a movement, have bridged the growing gaps in abortion access for decades, standing up for providers and patients when it seemed like no one else would. Without them, access to safe, legal abortion would have disappeared long before the crisis moment in which America now finds itself. Their story has never been told—until now.

• • •

This book isn't a legal dissection of *Roe v. Wade* or any other abortion-related law, nor is this a dissection of what the Supreme Court did in *Dobbs v. Jackson Women's Health Organization*. This book was written before *Roe* was struck down, before a leaked draft of the opinion exploded across the world in May 2022. Many marginalized folks were already living in a more or less post-*Roe* world prior to *Dobbs*, where some people already had to drive hundreds of miles to get to a clinic. In this moment, faced with an acute human rights crisis in the United States, I believe that what will help get us out of this terrifying, draconian mess isn't conjecture, but action.

The reason that abortion access has hobbled along for as long as it has isn't because *Roe v. Wade* is sacrosanct, but because everyday people stood up and found a way to make it a reality. A significant reason why legal abortion has largely remained accessible, from the years of bombing to the era of bans, is because of clinic escorts.

Whenever I put on my neon vest and started another morning shift as a clinic escort, I didn't spend my time wondering how a federal judge would rule on the latest abortion restriction, or about the balance of the Supreme Court. I couldn't do that. My role wouldn't allow me to. Instead, I had to respond to the immediacy of the person in front of me, to their body language, their words, their breath. I had to focus on the humanity of the person I was serving. I had to support them in a moment of need.

At its core, volunteering as a clinic escort isn't about politics or pontificating. It's about responding, as a human being, to another human being's needs. It's about dignity, compassion, and kindness. It's about people. It's that commitment that can light the way for all of us to approach abortion not as a caustic political fight but as a matter of human dignity, no matter how you personally feel about abortion. Even without *Roe v. Wade*, there is profound power in that, if we choose to take it.

Clinic escorts have put their bodies on the line for other people, for other people's choices, their bodies, their lives. They have shown up despite bombs, bans, shootings, and a global pandemic to support patients and providers, to keep safe abortion accessible. Safe, legal abortion is only a memory if we allow it to become one. This is the story of how everyday people have, for decades, refused to let that happen.

One

The Birth of a Movement

IT WAS ALREADY NEARING EIGHTY DEGREES IN THE EARLY morning hours of August 2, 1975, when a small group convened outside Sigma Reproductive Health Services, the only abortion clinic in Rockville, Maryland.[1] Orchestrated by Burke Balch and former antiwar activist Thomas Mooney, six women entered the clinic under the guise of being patients. Once inside, they sat down and refused to move.

Women were the only protesters to occupy the space, an attempt by the male organizers to defuse any claims of misogyny. While inside, the women sang songs and led prayers for the unborn. Outside, the male organizers preached, handed out literature, and called to every patient who went inside, pleading with them to turn around and forgo abortion. Clinic staff were caught off guard and patients had no idea what was going on around them. Eventually, the police were called and the six women were arrested.[2]

It was the first antiabortion sit-in in American history. No one at Sigma Reproductive Health Services that day could have predicted what this singular protest would spawn in the decades to come, a movement whose willingness to end abortion at any and all costs would not only pave the way for the possible end of *Roe v. Wade*—it would also lead to murder.

• • •

On January 22, 1973, Carol Downer's phone rang while she was enjoying a much-needed day off from the women's health center where she worked in Los Angeles. She strolled over to the phone, in no particular hurry. She was going to savor the day away from work.

For the past four years, she had worked herself to the bone. After attending a meeting of the National Organization for Women, Betty Friedan's new women's rights organization, in 1969, Downer devoted herself to the effort to legalize abortion, an outgrowth of the women's liberation movement. Downer herself had had two illegal abortions, and she knew firsthand how important access to safe abortion was to women's autonomy and equality.

By the time Downer experienced her unplanned pregnancies, abortion had been illegal in the United States for nearly a century. But for much of the nineteenth century, abortion was legal until the point of "quickening," the point at which the pregnant person can feel the fetus move, well into the second trimester. As abortion was largely performed by midwives and homeopaths, the move to criminalize it coincided with a consolidation of power by doctors and medical professionals of the day. By the end of the century, legal abortion was a mere memory. By 1967, abortion had been decriminalized in Colorado, Oregon, North Carolina, and Downer's home state of California, but only a very few abortions were permitted for extenuating circumstances. In 1970, Hawaii made history as the first state to legalize abortion at the request of the pregnant person. New York shortly followed suit, and the few states that had legal abortion began to serve as de facto hubs for those who were financially able to get there. But that still meant that most people who sought an abortion wouldn't be able to legally get one. For those determined to have one, that often meant risking their lives.

Downer's illegal abortions were safe, but she knew how lucky she was to be alive. In 1930, just three years before Downer was born, abortion—then illegal nationwide—was listed as the official cause of death for 2,700 people, nearly one in five maternal deaths. By 1965, when Downer was on the verge of her new life as an abortion activist, the number of deaths from illegal and unsafe abortion had fallen, but still accounted for 17 percent of maternal deaths.[3] Unless performed by a trained and experienced person, illegal abortion could be outright deadly.

Downer not only became an outspoken advocate for legalized abortion; she also joined fellow activists in making safe underground abortion possible. In 1969, the health center where she worked began covertly referring pregnant people to trusted doctors who would provide safe yet clandestine abortions. Before *Roe* legalized abortion, Downer's group had a cohesive structure in place to make safe abortion accessible. "We already had an abortion referral service [through] the women's center and we gave [patients] an exam to see how far along they were. We [then] scheduled them at a small accredited hospital near us that we had made contact with to reserve a small set of operating rooms, and we had hired a doctor [to perform the abortions]."

The same year that Downer's group began referring patients to physicians for covert abortions, a group of feminists in Chicago, Illinois, set out on a similar path. The Abortion Counseling Service of Women's Liberation began by referring patients to a small group of reliable doctors who would secretly provide abortions. Signs went up all over the city: PREGNANT? DON'T WANT TO BE? CALL JANE, along with a telephone number. The Jane Collective, as it came to be known, soon decided to take matters into their own hands—literally. They learned from one of the doctors, firsthand, how to safely perform abortions themselves. In their four-year existence, they performed thousands of safe, illegal abortions.

Downer's group was on the same trajectory. Their mission wasn't just to make safe underground abortion possible, but to support everyone who went through that experience. "We took these women—we accompanied them and counseled them . . . We went with them and helped them get through the experience. We already had contact with doctors. We already knew the procedure. We'd learned it ourselves!"[4]

By 1973, years of activism and an escalating feminist movement made Downer hopeful. "I certainly predicted that the walls were coming down," she said to me in a matter-of-fact tone. "I could see it . . . it was in the air. [We knew] that abortion was going to get legalized, but we didn't realize [when] or how much."

When Downer answered the phone on that January day in 1973, she got her answer—the time was now. In the landmark ruling *Roe v. Wade*, the Supreme Court of the United States of America legalized abortion nationwide. The Court made it clear: the decision to have an abortion was between the pregnant person and her doctor, not the government.

"I was taken aback," Downer recalled. "I was happy as could be!" What began as a day off became a celebration, calling friends and fellow activists all day long. The ruling was more than most of them even thought possible. Rather than a gradual extension of abortion to select patients, it was now unconstitutional for states to restrict abortion *for anyone at all*. Abortion would have to be legal in every state at least to the point of "fetal viability," the point at which the fetus can theoretically survive outside the womb (typically twenty-four to twenty-eight weeks).

Within a matter of minutes, everyone in every state had a constitutional right to an abortion.

• • •

Roe was transformative. Freestanding clinics began to sprout across states where abortion had been criminalized for more than a century. At the beginning of the 1970s, abortion was legal in only a few states and under the most extreme situations. By the end of the decade, there were 459 clinics across the country, all dedicated to providing safe abortion care.[5] In 1985, after a dozen years of legalization, 87 percent of abortions were performed in freestanding clinics, replacing hospitals as the go-to location for safe abortion care.[6]

Those clinics, created as safe havens that specialized in a unique and newly legal form of health care, weren't prepared for the growing antiabortion hostility. The swiftness with which abortion became legalized nationwide helped trigger the emergence of a powerful, committed antiabortion movement, one determined to overturn *Roe* at any cost. The sit-in protest that occurred in Rockville, Maryland, was only the beginning. Clinic staff and providers had no idea what was awaiting them.

• • •

In June 1978, Susan Hill had done the unthinkable—she'd finally opened an abortion clinic in Fort Wayne, Indiana. Nearly a year after its mayor defiantly declared that "this clinic will never open," after months of negotiations, regulations, and permit disputes, the Fort Wayne Women's Health Organization (FWWHO) was finally able to see patients.[7] The thrill of victory wouldn't last long.

Protesters began to gather out front within days. "Are you going to kill your baby?" they would scream at patients walking into the clinic. One of the protesters, an ex-Benedictine monk from Chicago named Joseph Scheidler, was there regularly, screaming into a bullhorn about the "child-killing industry" and the "culture of death" that went on inside.[8] Some of his fellow protesters even grabbed patients' arms and elbows to get their attention, refusing to let them pass until they pried their arm away or a staff member saw what was happening and managed to intervene.[9]

At one point, two protesters intercepted a twelve-year-old girl and her fifteen-year-old sister. They took the teenagers three blocks away to a nearby McDonald's, gave the twelve-year-old a pregnancy test, and erroneously told her that she wasn't pregnant. They talked to the girls about abortion, describing it in graphic detail and calling it murder. When the girls' mother found out, she was apoplectic. She already knew about her daughter's pregnancy; because she had to work that day, she had asked her eldest daughter to take her pregnant daughter to the clinic.[10] The twelve-year-old was eventually able to have her abortion.

Desperate to avoid another incident like that, Hill and the staff of FWWHO accepted a local feminist group's offer to help walk patients past the protesters and safely into the clinic. A spry, spiky-haired woman named Ann Horn was one of them. Recruited by a friend, she came to the clinic one Sunday and stood, filling with anger, as protesters called the patients entering the clinic "baby killers." At one point, one of the protesters pulled her aside and said, "I hope I catch you in a dark alley."[11]

"I heard some of the things they were saying to the women," she said. "I couldn't *not* go back."

On August 11, 1979, the clinic had a waiting room full of patients and an entrance filled with protesters. Scheidler, wielding his bullhorn, joined the nearly three dozen protesters outside, some of whom had shown up as early as midnight to begin their siege. He shouted at women walking into the clinic: "Your cervix will be cracked!" "What kind of mother will your children think you are when they learn you killed their brother and sister?"

Inside, the phone rang. It was a bomb threat, the clinic's first.

After a security guard told them the harrowing news, the escorts hurried to the back door to help patients evacuate. As staff and patients emerged, escorts came to greet them, only to realize that the protesters were right on their heels. On the spot, staff and escorts devised a plan: the staff ushered patients and their relatives to a park across the street and the escorts formed a circle around them. It did little to deter Scheidler and his fellow protesters, who tried everything from yelling at and photographing patients to attempting to physically break through the escorts' human shield.[12]

The police did nothing. The city refused to dispatch either police or fire officials. A bomb squad technician answered the call but refused to search the clinic because he was "unfamiliar with the contents." Instead, the clinic staff were forced to search for the potential bomb themselves while clinic escorts protected patients with their bodies.[13] Mercifully, there was no bomb to be found that day.

"We were on our own and we knew it," Horn recalled.

It was the very early days of clinic escorting. There was no formal training. There were no materials on how to handle harassment and keep your cool. These early volunteers had no idea that they were among the first ever to embark on something like this—they just knew it had to be done.

Horn and her fellow escorts, that tiny handful of feminists in very conservative Fort Wayne, had to learn from experience how to be aware of their surroundings and how to deescalate a potentially volatile situation. They learned how to use their bodies as shields to deflect the screams and body checks from the increasingly hostile protesters that swarmed the front door. Their team began to line up in front of the clinic door to keep protesters from rushing it or blocking the entrance, only to find that this gave protesters the length of the sidewalk to follow and harass patients. They were pioneers, figuring it out as they went, hoping to just get the next patient in the door and keep the clinic open for another day.

The skills they honed in those early years would serve them well as the seventies became the eighties, because things were about to get much worse.

The Opposition Escalates

By 1983, *Roe v. Wade* had been the law of the land for a decade. Abortion opponents always believed that the longer it remained in place, the harder it would be to overturn. Every year that passed since *Roe*'s decision put their goal further out of reach. Trying to shut down abortion clinics became even more critical to their ultimate goal.

The peaceful sit-in and sing-along in the reception area of Sigma Reproductive Health Services was now a distant memory. Acts of vandalism and violence were more commonplace. By the end of 1983, there had been more than twenty bombings and arson attacks against abortion clinics,[14] and a new antiabortion terrorist group, calling itself the "Army of God," even kidnapped an abortion provider along with his wife.[15] For clinic staff, doing their job now meant accepting the very real possibility of harm.

In response, some clinics began to use volunteer escorts. The National Organization for Women (NOW) and some of its local affiliates helped to organize volunteers in cities and towns where clinics were under increasing threat.

When Patricia Baird-Windle's Aware Woman Center for Choice

clinic moved from Cocoa Beach to nearby Melbourne, Florida, in 1982, she asked police for help with the growing aggression from protesters. After the officers told her they could do nothing in response to a protester screaming for hours on end, she had had enough. "From then on I had NOW people at the clinic as patient escorts."[16]

By May 1983, Planned Parenthood League of Massachusetts (PPLM) was dealing with daily confusion from patients who couldn't distinguish between the actual Planned Parenthood clinic and the antiabortion pregnancy center Problem Pregnancy that went by the deceptive name of PP Inc., located in the same building. Protesters would line the hallways of the building and sow such turmoil and terror for patients that PPLM eventually brought in volunteer clinic escorts to stand in the hallways and direct patients to the real clinic so they wouldn't miss their appointments.[17]

In Philadelphia, picketing got so bad at the Northeast Women's Center that Mary Banneker, the clinic administrator, decided to do the same. She contacted the northeast chapter of NOW and asked them to recruit clinic escorts to walk patients and staff past the picketers. Soon, clinic escorts were out in front of the clinic, trying to shield patients from the vitriol as they escorted them to the front door. But within a few weeks, the situation outside Northeast Women's Center became untenable. Finally, the clinic pulled the plug on the escort team after an escort was violently shoved into a bush by an antiabortion protester.[18] Banneker and staff were unwilling to continue to risk the health and safety of their volunteers.

• • •

In January 1984, Katherine Taylor was recovering from surgery in her hometown of Portland, Oregon, when she realized she was pregnant. Fearful of the possible impact that carrying the pregnancy to term could have on her health and the health of the fetus, she decided to have an abortion. She told her boyfriend and her family, who immediately rallied behind her. Her mother, Joy, aware of the growing protests at Portland Feminist Women's Health Center, where Katherine had scheduled her abortion, insisted that they all accompany her to the appointment.

When they pulled up that January afternoon, they saw twelve men and one woman holding court outside the clinic.

"As I approached the picketers, they became louder and more obnoxious," Katherine told the House Subcommittee on Civil and Constitutional Rights in a hearing on antiabortion violence in 1985.[19] "They started yelling things at me like 'Two lives go in and one comes out! Baby killer! Murderer!' Each sign they were holding had the word 'Murderer' written on it."

One man screamed in Joy's face, "Baby killer!" The only female picketer bellowed "Auschwitz" over and over.

The Taylor family had a plan to insulate Katherine as much as possible—her brother and boyfriend flanked either side of her while her mother and father brought up the front and the rear. They walked that way, as a bubble of protection around her, until they got in the door.

Without realizing it, the Taylor family became temporary clinic escorts that day, surrounding Katherine on all sides to serve as a physical and emotional buffer.

"I was very fortunate compared to the other women that go to the clinic because I had my family with me," she testified. "They could get to my brother or anyone else in my family, but they couldn't touch me. The other women that go in there, they don't have that. All the girls that were in my group, they did not have anyone to come with. They had to face those picketers by themselves and go through that picket line with no one."

While clinic escorts were emerging at some clinics and disappearing from others, by 1984 many clinics still didn't have any. More state and local NOW chapters began providing escort services to clinics in need, but this was done on a mostly ad hoc basis, with no real organizational structure.[20] Some abortion providers worried that having clinic escorts would actually inflame tensions by goading antiabortion activists into bringing even bigger numbers to their front doors. Without anyone like Ann Horn dedicated to supporting patients at other clinics, staff and patients were left to navigate the increasing volatility and, in some places, outright danger on their own.

• • •

As the feminist volunteers in Fort Wayne were learning on the job, so were their protesters. Joe Scheidler, the bullhorn-wielding ex-monk who cut his chops outside FWWHO, took what he learned and formalized it across the state line in his hometown of Chicago.

He founded the Pro-Life Action League (PLAL) in 1980, a direct-action initiative that pioneered some of the most relentless and lasting antiabortion protest tactics in the country, including individualized and targeted harassment. At one point in 1982, Scheidler learned of an eleven-year-old girl who was scheduled to have an abortion at a local Chicago hospital. According to the *Chicago Tribune*, "He located the child's residence through a private detective and then, unannounced, went to an apartment balcony next to that of the girl's family, and using his longtime companion, a Radio Shack bullhorn, harangued her mother, demanding to see the child alone. The mother refused."[21]

In 1985, Scheidler published *Closed: 99 Ways to Stop Abortion*, which systematized many of the then haphazard and disparate antiabortion protest activities. In it, he detailed an extensive list of harassment techniques designed to force clinics to close, including how to track motor vehicle information of patients and how to render a clinic's telephone lines inoperable with a flood of calls.[22] He also emphasized the importance of "sidewalk counseling," a misnomer for the kind of direct, in-your-face contact that he had horrifyingly attempted with the pregnant eleven-year-old girl three years earlier.

At this time, most Chicago-area clinics lacked escorts or even basic security.[23] And Scheidler was a showman, using his media prowess to develop connections in the fervently antiabortion Reagan administration that solidified his status as "untouchable" by law enforcement. By 1986, Scheidler was a bona fide star in the antiabortion movement. Revered for his willingness to openly flout trespassing laws and his abrasive, tenacious style that earned him the nickname "the Green Beret of the pro-life movement" from Pat Buchanan—then the communications director for the Reagan White House—Scheidler was the central figure of antiabortion protest and resistance. PLAL's meetings became a unique chance for abortion opponents to radicalize, learn new tactics, and network. It was at their annual conference in April of that year in St. Louis that Randall Terry, an ex–used car salesman and aspiring fanatic, would meet his mentor. A new era of mass pandemonium at clinics was about to begin.

• • •

By the time he met Scheidler, Randall Terry had already flirted with direct action and illegal protest activity, harassing patients at Southern Tier Women's Center in his hometown of Binghamton, New York.[24] But meeting Scheidler fueled Terry's desire for grandeur and his willingness to violate the law in new ways. With the help of his role model and mentor, Terry created a new antiabortion organization called Operation Rescue.

Unlike its predecessors, Operation Rescue wasn't interested in simply protesting abortion clinics; it wanted to shut them down entirely. Terry and his followers would stop clinics from operating by literally blocking entrances, inundating them with hundreds of bodies,[25] and doing everything from putting glue in the locks to chaining themselves to the front doors or to the lab equipment inside.[26] They called these blockades "rescues."

The organization's tactics, eschewed by some mainstream antiabortion organizations, turned the front door of a clinic into a carnival of chaos.[27] The results were devastating. Rather than dealing with one-off or more localized incidents of harassment, clinics now dealt with a growing machine, funded by heavyweights like Jerry Falwell's Moral Majority, that refused to even pretend that it adhered to the law.[28] Operation Rescue would target cities they felt were vulnerable or prime for a major media moment, bring in hundreds or even thousands of protesters from out of town, and descend on a clinic that was, most likely, independently owned and without any real structural support. Emboldened by Scheidler and willing to endure jail time, Operation Rescue protesters were willing to physically tussle to shut down a clinic.

Veteran activist Sue Davis noticed the shift. Most of the earlier antiabortion protesters had declared themselves pacifists. "They'd try to hand out brochures and they didn't really do a lot of chanting. They were more passive," she explained. "But Operation Rescue was not passive. They were hateful."[29]

"Rescues" began taking place in cities across the country. Terry led his first massive solo "rescue" at Cherry Hill Women's Center in Cherry Hill, New Jersey, on November 28, 1987. Three hundred protesters flew in from nineteen other states at their own expense to be trained by Terry in civil disobedience for "the unborn." Terry and his fanatical flock descended on the clinic early that morning, sealing off access to the building and halting abortion services.[30] By day's end, more than two hundred of them were arrested in the first successful mass blockade of an abortion clinic.[31]

In 1988, Operation Rescue conducted 182 blockades,[32] one of which resulted in the arrests of more than 1,600 protesters for blockading offices of the National Organization for Women and Planned Parenthood in New York City.[33]

But the abortion rights movement was learning, too. Capitalizing on the Pope's visit to Detroit in the fall of 1987, Scheidler and Terry teamed up to wreak havoc on the city's abortion clinics. In response, local citizens and national abortion rights activists got together to develop one of the first clinic defense networks in the country. The nonexistent response from law enforcement, whose efforts were directed at protecting the Pope, left Detroit's abortion rights community to figure out a way to keep the clinics open all on their own. NARAL's Judith Widdicombe headed to Detroit to train members of the Michigan Organization for Human Rights to be clinic escorts, coordinating with clinic staff on a strategy to keep the clinics open. Unlike previous clinic escort groups, which were isolated and learning as they went, Detroit's new cohort was trained specifically to respond to the anticipated blockade.

At six o'clock on the morning of the Pope's visit, the newly trained clinic escorts fanned out to the twenty-one (of Detroit's twenty-four) abortion clinics that had decided to open their doors that day. When Scheidler's activists descended on Summit Medical Center, "the group clashed with forty escorts who formed human shields and walked women into the clinic, amid jeers and picket signs," reported *The Detroit News*.[34] Eventually, police responded and arrested twenty protesters.[35] Every single one of the clinics that opened their doors that morning saw patients that day.

In the summer of 1988, Terry decided to target abortion clinics during the Democratic National Convention in Atlanta, Georgia, unveiling what he called "The Siege of Atlanta."[36] Almost immediately, abortion clinics across Atlanta tried to prepare. They organized a shared space where patients could go to wait, in case of blockades at a given clinic. Clinic escorts offered to fan out and move as needed.[37]

Dianne Mathiowetz, a forty-two-year-old auto worker living in Atlanta, had been active in social justice causes for nearly two decades. As a graduate student at the University of Virginia in the early 1970s, she helped pave the way for the eventual legalization of advertising abortion services when she, as a member of the *Virginia Weekly* underground newspaper and in violation of Virginia's restrictive law, included information on how to obtain legal abortion services in New York State. Mathiowetz and her newspaper's boss, Jeff Bigelow, refused to let the law stand, and in 1975 it was struck down by the Supreme Court in *Bigelow v. Virginia*, just two years after *Roe*.

Now, Mathiowetz brought her swagger and determined commitment to the Feminist Women's Health Center in Atlanta, where she quickly learned what Operation Rescue could do to a clinic and the patients it served.

"The clinics were really under attack psychologically, physically," Mathiowetz said. Operation Rescue, buoyed by a national recruitment effort led by the Christian Broadcasting Network, brought in protesters by the busload.

> The task was to greet a client and there'd be a couple of us, and we'd be around this woman. We first asked her, did she want us to help her get into the clinic? Because it was intimidating with these mostly [male], very hostile crowds and all the signs they had of fetuses and stuff like that, horrible things about women being murderers and stuff. We would essentially use an umbrella or our coat or shawl and kind of

help this woman get out of her car, hopefully not be facially
identified [by the picketers], and get her into the building.[38]

But there was only so much a clinic escort could do if the clinic
was blockaded. "To some degree, abortion opponents were across
the street, but a lot of times they were on the sidewalk, with just a
little bit of space in front of the building," she said. "[And there was]
no real police support, in my opinion."[39]

It would last for the entire summer. By the end, Mathiowetz
and her fellow clinic escorts were utterly exhausted and infuriated,
and more than 1,300 Operation Rescue protesters would end up in
handcuffs, including Terry himself.[40]

He was just getting started.

A Burgeoning Battleground

By the time the "Siege of Atlanta" was over, Terry's plan had worked:
Operation Rescue was a national name. The number of protesters swelled, alongside the number of arrests. Terry made the media rounds, everything from Pat Robertson's Christian Broadcasting
Network to *The Oprah Winfrey Show*.[41] Operation Rescue blockades
were featured on every imaginable news program, from *60 Minutes*[42]
to *NBC Evening News*.[43] The number of rescues continued to escalate, and Terry became more determined to shut down more clinics,
all while growing his own national brand.

It was painful for many clinic staff to see Terry, a man who had
committed to making their lives hell, validated on national television. Here was a man who openly flouted the law, who oversaw
some of the most egregious forms of targeted harassment of abortion
providers, who gleefully shut down their clinics with the bodies of

hundreds of loyal, fanatical supporters. Every media appearance must have felt like a taunt.

But over time, the media blitz also helped galvanize and motivate those on the other side of the issue as well. Abortion clinic harassment and violence wasn't a mainstream topic in 1988. The outgoing Reagan administration was openly antiabortion, even inviting Joseph Scheidler, Terry's mentor, to the White House.[44] Subcommittees in the House of Representatives had held a few small hearings on this issue, but it was, for the most part, invisible to much of the American public—until Operation Rescue forced them to see what was happening.

Up until this point, clinic escorts were largely passive, typically avoiding engagement with the protesters and focusing solely on the patient. But once Operation Rescue started shutting down clinics, some abortion rights supporters felt that nonengagement was no longer enough.

For the most part, law enforcement was scattered, disorganized, or even apathetic. Most weren't prepared to deal with the onslaught of bodies that parked themselves directly in front of clinics, and since most of those bodies were white and middle-class, law enforcement seemed to give them a bit more leeway than they did other groups. At a clinic in San Francisco, law enforcement waited two hours before even beginning to arrest hundreds of blockaders at the Pregnancy Consultation Center, forcing clinic staff and patients to wait outside amid the melee while the doors remained blocked.[45]

This was intolerable to local activists. By 1988, the Bay Area, long home to radicals and the counterculture, became a hub for a new kind of activist movement: clinic defense. These activists combined traditional clinic escorting with more physical defensive tactics to keep Operation Rescue from blockading their clinics and shutting down abortion access. They called themselves the Bay Area Coalition Against Operation Rescue (BACAOR).

BACAOR's philosophy was bold and brash. "Our first line of defense for protection of reproductive rights is self-defense. We cannot rely on the courts, police, or legislatures to protect our fundamental rights to control our bodies and reproductive options."

BACAOR set up a central office with multiple phone lines to coordinate defense for the many clinics across the Bay Area. They had a formal reporting structure, with clinic defense captains who oversaw strategy and tactics on site. Every defender was expected to be at their assigned clinic no later than 5:30 a.m. to ensure they were there before Operation Rescue arrived. They designated some members as traditional escorts, whose jobs were focused on finding and supporting patients as they walked what was often a gauntlet.[46] They even had opposition trackers, who would follow cars and attempt to infiltrate Operation Rescue.

"We trusted each other, and we gave each other really good information," recalled Angela Bocage, who was a member of BACAOR for a year during its heyday. "We had people willing to be out there early and do what was necessary and a 'do what it takes' attitude. Not waiting for law enforcement or city council or whatever because nothing was helping, it was just a great PR show for people who hated women. They were just cruel."[47]

Unlike other groups, BACAOR was not afraid to get physical. Their informational pamphlet made clear what newbie defenders could expect: "We emphasize that we are there to defend ourselves and to defend the clinic, and that we can expect to go away with bruises or sore muscles if [Operation Rescue] hits there." If they felt they had to, they would physically move or restrain Operation Rescue protesters in order to get a patient in the door.[48]

They even got creative with ways to keep the protesters from rushing the door. Several defenders would stand by the door. In front of them, a row of defenders would stand side-by-side, holding pieces of plywood that they called "defense boards," essentially making a wall to keep Operation Rescue out. On the other side of the wall were four designated "rovers," who were tasked with watching the opposition. During one blockade, "when the first client and her boyfriend arrived, our four 'rovers' signaled to those behind the boards which end we intended to break, then we had a huddle, decided which [protesters] to go for, and went straight to them, pulling [them] out of place while the client and her boyfriend went through. The defenders at the door opened up one of the defense boards and the client got in behind it."[49]

They were unlike any other clinic escort team, and they got results.

BACAOR defenders were credited with "the effect of decreasing the numbers of 'casual blockaders' who participated in the early stages," a not-insignificant victory that illuminated that showing up and standing defiantly in defense of the clinics could help stem the tide of the insidious and growing blockades.[50]

As a result, BACAOR's tactics quickly spread across the country.

In Washington, D.C., a loose coalition developed, centered around the explicit goal of keeping D.C.-area abortion clinics open and Operation Rescue as far from the entrances as possible. They called themselves the Washington Area Clinic Defense Task Force (WACDTF), and they utilized both traditional clinic escort and some of the newer clinic defense tactics that BACAOR was pioneering out west.

WACDTF pioneered the integration of clinic escorting and clinic defense. "[It was] not a bright line of the two categories, but two ends of a log," said Alicia Lucksted, who has been with WACDTF since 1989. She recalled how escorts and defenders would work together during a blockade to allow patients to get inside.

You have that amount of [defenders] at the door, and other [defenders] maybe could be standing around the side of the wall of the building that goes out to the sidewalk. If we could manage that, either beforehand or as the blockade progressed, then you can use yourself as a buffer, so if there's people lining the wall and they could all step out a few feet, the way behind them would be a corridor . . . Sometimes, we were indeed able to have access to a clinic or preserve access by just making these bubbles of space. Then other people, in a formal escorting role . . . might actually see somebody come up and they could say, "Hey, this is the situation, there's all these people being very loud and obnoxious. We have this wall of people who are linking arms and you can walk behind them and against the wall. The clinic is open and safe and okay."[51]

Ann Horn and her compatriots in Fort Wayne, Indiana, were already a decade into keeping their clinic open when Operation Rescue came on the scene. What had once seemed as bad as it could be was now child's play—at one point, five thousand Operation Rescue protesters descended on the clinic.[52] But the clinic also had a community of supporters; at one point more than 350 people were on-site to defend it.[53] Horn recalled how she and her fellow escorts prepared for an upcoming blockade in the late 1980s with a homemade plywood fence, inspired by the clinic defenders in BACAOR:

I remember standing about a block away. We were watching for them because we knew they were coming . . . We heard the cry go up from the clinic and we sprinted back. That clinic was on very small property, city sidewalk and a park next door so they could get really close. There was no way we were going to get a fence [from law enforcement]. We made a fence. If you were on the inside of that fence, you had to be prepared to be there for a while. They were kicking us and we just had to use all of our strength. Some [of us] were sitting down with our arms locked and others were holding up from the top. And it was constant pressure, physical pressure, kicking at us. Verbally berating us. It was really hard because we were committed to nonviolence, and that was hard. That was hard through all of that. We did that for hours and got women in, got staff in, passed them up over the fence until enough of [the protesters were] arrested. Then we went home all battered and sore and hungry and thirsty.

Neighboring Ann Arbor, Michigan, a hub for the radical student left in the late 1960s, had its own clinic defense group. In the spring of 1989, Danielle Lescure was a twenty-one-year-old recent college graduate when she joined her friend for a meeting of the Ann Arbor Committee to Defend Abortion Rights. Within the hour, she became a clinic defender.

That summer, Lescure and her fellow defenders would try to figure out which Ann Arbor clinic Operation Rescue was targeting. Some days they would get there first and form a line, arms linked, across the front of the clinic. Lescure and others would seek out patients and shuffle them past the line of defenders while Operation Rescue protesters were pushing in from the outside. Most of the time they were unsuccessful, getting to the clinic after a blockade was already in place, and the clinic would have to close for the day.

One hot summer morning, Lescure and her fellow defenders showed up too late once again. About one hundred Operation Rescue protesters were occupying both the front and the back entrances;

no one could get in or out. A parking lot across the street was filled with patients in their cars, waiting to get into their now delayed appointments. The clinic, a standalone one-story building, appeared to be shuttered, when a staff member noted a window around the other side of the building into which she could crawl. On the fly, the clinic staff and defenders came up with a novel idea: the side window could become an entrance.

"There'd be a few of us [defenders] shielding [the patient] and making our way, as casually as possible, across the street [from the parking lot]," Lescure remembered. "Then there were a few discreetly, casually by the window so no one would notice. And then we were sneaking her in that way. The clinic staff was in there and they could help them through the window."[54]

Lescure and her fellow defenders felt euphoric that day. They had managed to keep the clinic open and had helped patients access abortion. But the fact was not lost on her that, more than sixteen years after *Roe v. Wade* was decided, a clinic in a liberal city like Ann Arbor had to covertly smuggle patients in through a side window, just to have a legal health-care procedure. And that was considered a victory, no less.

• • •

In New York City, Mary Lou Greenberg was searching for both a community and a way to fight back against Operation Rescue when she came upon the New York Pro-Choice Coalition, an emerging group of activists and clinic staff dedicated to promoting abortion rights. Founded in 1985 by New York icon and abortion care pioneer Merle Hoffman, it took the lead in responding to Operation Rescue's planned blockade of New York City clinics from April 30 to May 7, 1988.[55]

Not everyone in the coalition was on board with clinic defense as a primary tactic, Greenberg remembered. She and others, including Hoffman, were adamant that something needed to be done. A stand needed to be taken, they argued. The clinic defense advocates won out, and they began developing a formal clinic defense strategy.[56]

Operation Rescue was following their usual playbook; while they had announced that they planned to blockade New York City abortion clinics, they deliberately didn't mention which ones. This would spread law enforcement and clinic escorts and defenders thin, forcing them to try to cover all of their bases at once.

Organizers began reaching out to every abortion clinic in New York City, alerting them to the impending "hit" and sharing security tips and strategies with them. Some clinics even became actively involved in defense planning with the coalition.[57]

Learning from BACAOR (who actually sent some activists to New York to help), the New York coalition immediately set up a formal structure with dedicated roles.[58] NOW served as "command central," and all orders came through their office to ensure alignment. They designated opposition watchers, people who would keep tabs on where the Operation Rescue protesters were staying and where they were going, as well as clinic watchers, whose job was to get to the clinics, sometimes as early as 3:00 a.m., and report into command central on the goings-on at their designated locations. Organizers created phone trees, automated telephone systems that would tell other clinic defenders where to go and when to get there. They worked with a friendly local radio station, WBAI, to disseminate information even more widely to supporters, particularly if the clinic had approved a counterdemonstration from abortion rights supporters. Notably, as in Fort Wayne, there were both escorts and defenders—some were tasked with walking patients and some were tasked with physically protecting the door.

One morning that week, Greenberg and the other defenders monitoring Operation Rescue were waiting outside a hotel in Times Square where they were known to be staying when protesters emerged from the front lobby. In the days before cell phones, there was no time to call in to central command from a nearby pay phone. They would have to follow them.

> We were right with them, running shoulder to shoulder with them. They went to the nearby subway, and the police were there, standing around. The police held the subway doors open, kept them open while all the "anti" people went in! We went inside at the same time but we were penned in with them, in the same car with a few police who weren't doing anything. But when they got out of the car, we knew we had to be there first. I remember running down the street to get to whatever clinic they were going . . . They had already gotten people who were massing, sitting there, and I remember seeing them. There were some police barricades trying to keep us penned into the other side of the street. But there were some of us who were not penned in and were trying to figure out how to get to the clinic doors, which had people sitting around it. There were some people who tried to dive in through this mass of people that were sitting down there. There was quite a bit of chaos there.

With the passive response from law enforcement, six hundred Operation Rescue protesters were able to blockade the clinic that day.[59] But clinic defenders didn't give up; they learned from what happened and got more adept at protecting clinics. As the week went on and Operation Rescue targeted other New York City abortion clinics, defenders became better at arriving early to prevent a full-fledged blockade. They worked with NARAL and NOW to demand a meeting with the New York City police commissioner about law enforcement's lackadaisical attitude toward Operation Rescue and to demand more protection for the clinics.[60] Most critically, they kept showing up.

"We felt strongly that no matter where they went, we had to gather too and do whatever we could not only to help patients get in but to have a pro-choice presence and just stop Operation Rescue, to expose to people what was going on and to call people out, to come out and defend the clinics," Greenberg explained. "Here were people on the streets, actually with their bodies, putting their bodies on the line, and saying, 'No, I'm not going let this go down without protesting this and doing everything I can to oppose it.'"

That show of defiance and defense would prove invaluable. As the world was about to see in Wichita, Kansas, without it, a clinic's existence was impossible.

• • •

Despite the successes that escorts and defenders were having, many clinics were still wary of or outright unwilling to have them. Worried that it would make the situation worse, some eschewed volunteer support at all.

Operation Rescue was also having issues of its own. While Randall Terry made the media rounds, some members were frustrated that, while Terry and the leaders of Operation Rescue continued to be bailed out of jail, many others were left with no financial or legal support. The summer of 1991 was a chance to signal their fortified return, their show of power and strength to the nation. Keith Tucci, the new executive director of Operation Rescue, announced a weeklong siege of abortion clinics in Wichita, Kansas, a "Summer of Mercy."

The staff at all three of Wichita's abortion clinics were well aware of the pandemonium they could expect. Dr. George Tiller, one of three Wichita providers and one of the only providers in the country who performed later abortions, had long been in the crosshairs of antiabortion protesters and vigilantes. In 1986, his clinic was nearly destroyed when a pipe bomb detonated.[61]

Law enforcement told Dr. Tiller that they couldn't guarantee access for patients. "I did not want to close but we struck a deal with the police," Dr. Tiller said in *Targets of Hatred*, which charts the rise of antiabortion violence and terrorism from the days before *Roe* up to 2000. "We would close for the week if they would guarantee us access to the clinic beginning the Sunday night of the week before Operation Rescue was supposed to come."[62] For one week, all three abortion clinics in Wichita would close, leaving it an abortion-free city for the first time since *Roe v. Wade* had been decided nearly two decades earlier.

It turned out to be a mistake, one that signaled to Operation Rescue and every wannabe antiabortion protester that even threatening to blockade a clinic would force its closure.[63] Word spread quickly among antiabortion organizations and phone hotlines that Wichita was abortion-free. This was their chance to make a statement by keeping it that way.[64]

As thousands of Operation Rescue supporters descended on Wichita, so did the camera crews. Tucci and his massive army of fanatics were everywhere, from nightly news segments to morning shows. In their minds, they had done it—they had stopped abortion in Wichita for the week. Once Operation Rescue saw the kind of press coverage they were getting amid their self-declared "success," they refused to stop. The original one-week siege now dragged on, as thousands more protesters flocked to the city and began escalating their tactics.

Once it reopened, the Wichita Women's Center opted for clinic escorts and defenders. "We had at least a few dozen, I would say," remembered Julie Burkhart, who spent her summer breaks from college working at the clinic. "They would have signs. They would dress up and sing silly songs. They were there to show support and to drive the antis away."

Burkhart and other staff members were even forced to spend the night at the clinic on more than one occasion that summer. They kept the doors open while clinic defenders helped deflect the aggression outside.[65]

Dr. Tiller opted to forgo clinic escorts and defenders. With the long-simmering hostility against him, his clinic became ground zero.

Just after eight o'clock on the morning of August 2, 1991, Dr. Tiller pulled his pickup truck up to the front of his clinic, as he did most mornings. But today was different. The gate to his clinic, which normally opened upon his arrival, was firmly closed. In front of it were hundreds of bodies, seated in arbitrary rows. "Stop killing babies!" they chanted. Dr. Tiller sat in the front seat of his truck, unable to move. His clinic was blockaded. Even he couldn't get inside, let alone the patients.[66]

Wichita police, including Chief Rick Stone, stood amid the mass of bodies, arms crossed, almost marveling at the situation. The crowd refused to disperse after Chief Stone gave a verbal warning. Eventually, police began to carry the limp bodies, one by one, away from the entrance of the clinic. By the time the way was clear, it was too late to open the clinic's doors for the day.

Eventually, after days of struggle, Tiller's clinic did open, but without escorts or defenders. Patients were forced to endure a gauntlet unlike anything seen before.

Sylvia Doe (not her real name) was one of them. The following year she testified before Congress about her harrowing experience at Dr. Tiller's clinic during the siege. Doe, pregnant with a nonviable fetus, traveled from the East Coast to Kansas for the procedure. It was hard enough for her, having to terminate a wanted pregnancy. But she told the House Subcommittee on Crime and Criminal Justice that what she endured from the Operation Rescue protesters was a "living nightmare."[67]

> We were told the next morning that we had to get in our cars and we had to line up, one after the other, in them, to wait while they arrested the people, that they wouldn't arrest these people or let us get access to the clinic unless we're actually there, and that, because we weren't able to get in, that they'd start to arrest them. We sat there for one whole day, in 109 degree heat, while about 1,600 people were swarming around our cars. They were screaming at us violently, spitting, pounding on the windows, holding huge, poster-sized pictures of bloody baby parts. It was [a] very volatile situation. I feared for my life.[68]

It took three days for Doe to finally be able to get into the clinic to have the abortion that she never even wanted to have in the first place.

Like Doe, every patient who approached the clinic was literally surrounded by a mob, forced to remain in their cars for hours. "Let it live," one woman screamed into the front window of a patient's car. "Let it be yours to suckle!" Eventually, protesters began to lie down in front of the patients' cars. Doe testified that she watched a man force a young child, screaming in fear, to lie in front of a moving car to stop it from approaching the clinic.[69]

Law enforcement, still going one by one to arrest and drag away the limp bodies of protesters, grew exhausted and frustrated. As soon as one person was arrested, another would take their place. Local news reported that at one point, city police had to use two city buses and a rental truck to haul away one day's worth of protesters from Dr. Tiller's clinic.[70]

After four weeks of anarchy at the clinics, and with the city's law enforcement utterly depleted, the federal government finally intervened. Federal judge Patrick F. Kelly took an almost unprecedented step when he called a national press conference to demand that Operation Rescue cease the blockades, threatening anyone who defied his order with arrest. "They should say farewell to their family and bring their toothbrush and I mean it because they're going to jail," he said of Terry, Tucci, and others.[71] Finally, he called in U.S. marshals to support law enforcement and keep the clinics open.[72]

Only then did the siege begin to wind down, finally ending after six brutal weeks. By the summer's end, 25,000 antiabortion protesters had flocked to Wichita[73] and more than 2,700 people had been arrested.[74] The city of Wichita became synonymous with Operation Rescue and rabid antiabortion protest, despite the fact that more than 60 percent of Wichita citizens strongly opposed the organization's tactics.[75] After that summer, Operation Rescue was no longer just a national name; it was now infamous, and ready for its next target.

• • •

In June 1992, New Yorker Moira Ariev felt like having a little fun. She had just finished a PhD program and desperately wanted to let loose for an evening. That night, she walked to Central Park from her Upper East Side apartment for an al fresco concert. As she entered the park, someone handed her a flyer that read KICK OPERATION RESCUE OUT OF NYC.[76] Moira had heard about the siege in Wichita the previous summer and was appalled. The flyer told supporters to come to the Friends Meeting House in the Stuyvesant neighborhood of Manhattan a week later to learn more.

The Friends Meeting House contained a large auditorium that could accommodate as many as a thousand people. That steamy July night, it was packed to the gills. Five thousand New Yorkers crammed into this mid-nineteenth-century building to learn how they could resist Operation Rescue and keep New York City's four dozen abortion clinics open by becoming clinic defenders.

One of those organizers was the veteran activist Sue Davis. She looked out at the thousands of faces and remembered how, just a few weeks earlier, she was shoulder to shoulder with thousands just like them in Buffalo, and how good it felt.

· · ·

Ellie Dorritie, a forty-nine-year-old mother and a longtime social justice activist, watched the Summer of Mercy coverage from her home in Buffalo, New York, in horror. Dorritie remembered what a pre-*Roe* world was like for women; she herself had had an illegal abortion, and while she was grateful that it was ultimately safe, she described the process of finding one "insulting and demeaning and degrading." She didn't want any other woman to ever have to go through what she went through to get an abortion.

"Wichita was not invisible to us," she remembered. "Everybody felt that defeat. Everybody felt the threat, and it *was* a threat."[77]

Dorritie had recently opened her home to Dianne Mathiowetz, whose job had been transferred to Buffalo in the fall of 1991.[78] Mathiowetz brought years of organizing and clinic escorting experience from Atlanta, which would serve her well in the months to come.

As 1991 became 1992, that threat for Ellie and Dianne became more acute: building upon the Summer of Mercy, Operation Rescue announced that they were coming to Buffalo for a "Spring of Life."

It wasn't Operation Rescue's first time in Buffalo—they had successfully blockaded clinics three years earlier in 1989. Hundreds were arrested for blocking entrance to the clinics, while "a local minister pulled what he claimed was an aborted fetus from a plastic container during a live radio show," according to *The New York Times*.[79] That minister turned out to be the Reverend Robert Schenck. Buffalo residents were happy to see Operation Rescue leave.

Now, they worried that their city would be the next Wichita,[80] particularly after their own mayor essentially welcomed Operation Rescue to town, saying, "If they can close down one abortion mill, then I think they'll have done their job."[81]

"We felt the primary problem in Wichita was that the response was not fast enough," Valerie Colangelo, a Buffalo resident who supported abortion rights, told *The Christian Science Monitor*.[82]

But Dorritie, Colangelo, and their fellow activists were determined that Buffalo would be a different story. They believed that they and they alone would have to be responsible for protecting the clinics and ensuring their ability to remain open. "Waiting for the cops to do it or the city government to do it was not going to happen," Dorritie told me. They knew that if they wanted to keep the clinics open and beat back the behemoth that was Operation Rescue, they were going to need more than determination: they were going to need bodies, and a lot of them.

Dorritie, Mathiowetz, and other local activists met in late January with a diverse coalition of social justice organizations, including the AIDS Coalition to Unleash Power (ACT UP), Women's Health Action and Mobilization (WHAM!), SUNY Women's Resource Center, the Media Coalition for Reproductive Rights, NOW, and others. Out of that meeting, Buffalo United for Choice (BUFC) was born. They developed a plan to keep the clinics open during the impending blockade.

"We didn't have the courts or the police to rely on," Dorritie said. "We had each other. [Operation Rescue was] coming in mid-April until mid-May to shut the clinics down for a month. We had an organization off the ground by mid-February."

BUFC was steadfast in its support for clinic defense. This ruffled some feathers. Some mainstream abortion rights organizations like the Pro-Choice Network weren't willing to support it as a tactic, afraid it would only embolden Operation Rescue, and some coalition members favored traditional tactics like contacting legislators.[83] Ultimately, the Pro-Choice Network left the coalition.[84]

Buffalo abortion providers, long suffering from a lack of support from law enforcement, were supportive of BUFC's efforts, which strengthened the coalition's commitment to clinic defense.[85] Within weeks, BUFC put out a call for clinic defense training. Dorritie worked closely with the Feminist Majority Foundation from California to train clinic defenders for the impending blockade.

"These sessions were, many times, hundreds of people in a big gymnasium or something, learning how to use their bodies to prevent some of the tactics of [Operation Rescue] people," Mathiowetz remembered. "It was really women getting ready for battle, they are battling for their rights and their lives."

Both organizations worked with local clinic escorts, long accustomed to the wild atmosphere at Buffalo clinic doors. "The patient escorts reviewed all the tactics to see how things would work and make it possible for us to help them to get patients safely into the

clinics," Dorritie said. "They certainly knew more about that than
we ever knew, and they were wonderful at being able to do that."[86]

By the time Operation Rescue finally came to Buffalo, BUFC
had trained up to six hundred clinic defenders.[87]

But BUFC did more than training; they developed an entire
self-contained system to protect the clinics. They knew that if it
was just about Buffalo, they would lose. They had learned from
other iterations of clinic defense groups that it was about more than
just showing up; they needed a structure and they needed visibility.
Dorritie remembers the huge undertaking:

> We put out countless press releases and called everybody.
> We had a hotline phone number. We had a P.O. box. We
> had calls from all over Buffalo and every other part of the
> United States, from people who wanted to join in, or help,
> or contribute, or write articles, or whatever they could do.
> We were on the *Today* show and *Nightline*, and we had a
> press committee. We did a national mailing, inviting people
> to come to Buffalo to defend the clinics. We printed some-
> thing like 150,000 leaflets and posters. We posted on every-
> thing that wasn't moving. We did fundraisers . . . We had
> equipment. We had walkie-talkies. We had a secret house
> with secret electrical reinforcement so we could charge these
> walkie-talkies. We had plants, people who were embedded
> in these right-wing churches, attending their meetings and
> planning.[88]

Mathiowetz, new to Buffalo but an old hat at organizing and
messaging, took on the role of national press officer. She made ap-
pearances on the *Today* show and CNN, and spoke with reporters at
nearly every imaginable national outlet. For the first time, Operation

Rescue wasn't allowed to unilaterally control the media narrative. With Mathiowetz at the wheel of national press, BUFC put out a clear and powerful message: this is about more than Buffalo; this is a national fight, and we need the nation to fight with us.[89]

As a result, everyone was going to Buffalo, it seemed. Ann Horn, by then a long-seasoned clinic escort and defender, traveled from Fort Wayne.[90] Mary Greenberg,[91] Sue Davis, and other members of the New York coalition made the road trip up north.[92] BACAOR sent clinic defenders as well, and the Feminist Majority Foundation brought hordes of young activists like duVergne Gaines, just a few years out of college but already an experienced clinic defender in Los Angeles. After what happened in Wichita, many were desperate for a chance to stand up to Operation Rescue and prove that there were people willing to protect abortion access.

The massive influx of clinic escorts and defenders made Buffalo unique, but that wasn't all. While it took four weeks for Judge Patrick Kelly to intervene and bring the federal marshals to Wichita, Buffalo abortion clinics shored themselves up from the beginning, obtaining an injunction from a federal judge that prohibited blockading the clinics. That gave law enforcement more clarity, and they began constructing barricades at clinics to keep protesters from the entrance. But this was Operation Rescue; they were used to violating the law and more than willing to get arrested.

Before dawn on the morning of Tuesday, April 21, 1992, fifteen hundred clinic defenders fanned out to the four Buffalo abortion clinics. By 5:00 a.m., every single door was covered, with defenders in position to protect the entrances from the impending blockades. Within an hour, Operation Rescue protesters were there, ready to wreak havoc and garner the same media attention that had rained down on them in Wichita.

Dorritie was at one of the clinics early that morning. As they got into formation, defenders could be heard chanting, "You're not in Kansas anymore!"[93] Dorritie and her fellow clinic defenders quickly linked both their arms and their legs, forming a barrier at the entrance and a small walkway through which escorts were able to guide patients. "There were so many of us, and we were so mouthy and so defiant and so *angry*," Dorritie said. "It was a real way for all of us to be able to express that, which had been without a channel for expression for a very long time. It was a blockade of a blockade!"[94]

Operation Rescue protesters, including Keith Tucci, tried to play a violent game of Red Rover with Dorritie and the clinic defense line, attempting to break through the human chain. "They look like zombies when they're trying to shut down a clinic and crawl through your physical bodies and the shields you're creating by linking arm to arm and shin to shin, and trying to keep these facilities open and safe and secure and protected from these extremists."

Time and again, they failed.

At Dr. Bart Slepian's suburban Buffalo clinic, Ann Horn was on deck, having flown in a few days earlier from Fort Wayne. Used to aggression and even physical jostling, she used her body, linked arm and arm, leg and leg with her fellow defenders, to reinforce the entrance and hold back Operation Rescue. Frustrated at their inability to break the defense line, protesters turned to physical aggression. "Some guy tried to pick me up and hurl me," Horn remembered. "There was this older African American man who had been at all of [the clinic defenses], Herb, and I heard him holler, 'Put her down!' and they dropped me like a sack of potatoes. They'd try to crawl under you and ram their heads into your crotch. We were so sore after Buffalo."[95]

Since they couldn't shut down any of Buffalo's clinics, protesters took to other forms of attention-seeking. At one point, the Reverend Robert Schenck, back in action in Buffalo, was arrested and charged with disorderly conduct for trying to shove a jar holding the remains of a nineteen-week-old fetus in the face of clinic defenders.[96]

One of the BUFC plants who successfully infiltrated Operation Rescue foiled their planned blockade one morning with a little deception. In line with their usual tactics, Operation Rescue leadership didn't announce the target until the morning of the blockade. But the anonymous BUFC infiltrator had gained their trust, pretending to be a member of their group for weeks. When they announced which clinic was up that morning, he offered to lead the caravan, since they were mostly from out of town. "He got them so damn lost, it took them an hour-plus before they figured out that they were just being led around Buffalo," Mathiowetz said. "So, they showed up at the clinic late, and some of them never made it at all." The defenders won again.[97]

About a week in, Operation Rescue leadership were aware of the impending public relations defeat, and so was BUFC. Having successfully infiltrated several local churches and working with opposition trackers from clinic defense groups across the country, BUFC knew exactly when the protesters planned to surge their protest, and they were ready for them, Dorritie recalled.

> About a week in, we had a big, crucial day where the pro-choice side of the siege was just huge and [Operation Rescue] was really determined that they were going to have a showdown. There were hundreds and hundreds and hundreds of people at the women's clinic. There were busloads of supporters from WHAM! that had come from NYC, carloads of people from you name it—Ithaca, Montreal, my daughter came from Boston with a busload of college women. The NOW National Board moved a national meeting from Tampa to Buffalo so that all their people would be

here. [Operation Rescue] was only able to put together 500 for that day and it was a really gorgeous sight. Not easily forgotten.[98]

By the time Operation Rescue left Buffalo in early May, the prevailing narrative that emerged was one of grassroots democracy in action and the power of the people to protect abortion clinics.

"A lot of women said it was life-changing when you were on the line," Mathiowetz said. "And it rained, I swear, every day, and we'd be out there at five o'clock, in front of these clinics, ankle-deep in mud, and nobody would leave. No matter how cold it got, no matter how wet you were, nobody would leave. I don't know if everybody perceived at the time how absolutely historic and how important they were, because after Buffalo, [Operation Rescue] lost their steam."

The media, which Mathiowetz expertly wielded, told the story of the siege that wasn't. "Though hundreds of anti-abortion protesters piled into Buffalo through the week, willing to go to jail to make their point, Operation Rescue did not shut down any abortions clinics here this week," reported *The New York Times*.[99] "No abortion clinics were closed, even for a minute," reported *The Buffalo News*.[100] According to United Press International, "Buffalo abortion rights advocates have staged the biggest and most organized resistance Operation Rescue has encountered."[101] And *Time* magazine was even more explicit about who won, declaring it "Operation Fizzle."[102]

It was a significant victory, one that NOW championed as its own.[103] But none of it would have been possible without everyday Buffalo residents like Ellie Dorritie and the scores of Americans who decided to speak out, stand up, and defend the clinics with their bodies. Two months later, Sue Davis would lead Moira Ariev and five thousand other New Yorkers in a defiant show of clinic defense,

shutting down every attempt by Operation Rescue to blockade the
city's clinics. Clinic escorting and clinic defense had gone mainstream by 1992, and the movement to beat back Operation Rescue
was gaining steam.

· · ·

By January 1993, *Roe v. Wade* had been settled law for two decades. It
had suffered a few judicial dents, including the 1992 Supreme Court
decision *Planned Parenthood v. Casey*, which upheld *Roe* but permitted
states to restrict abortion before the point of fetal viability as long as
they didn't place an "undue burden" on people seeking abortions.
But with Bill Clinton's inauguration, the first time in twelve years a
Democrat had occupied the White House, many clinic escorts and
defenders felt like the wind was finally at their backs rather than in
their faces.

"After Clinton was elected, everybody had a sense of forward
momentum," said Moira Ariev, who had taken the directive on that
flyer she was handed—to stop Operation Rescue—and run with it
as a clinic escort and defender in New York City.[104]

In Pittsburgh, Laura Horowitz, two years into her time as a
clinic escort and defender, felt much the same: "When Clinton came
in, we felt like [Operation Rescue was] very seriously demoralized."

If their dwindling number of activities and participants was any
indication, Operation Rescue certainly felt demoralized. By the end
of 1993, they were managing barely two dozen clinic blockades a
year, a shadow of their former power.[105] Many take credit for the decline and eventual disappearance of clinic blockades—abortion clinics and national organizations began filing injunctions to give the
clinics temporary relief from the onslaught of hundreds of protesters; law enforcement in Buffalo learned from failures in Wichita and

acted more decisively; and the changing political winds that ushered in a Democratic president certainly helped.

But all of those actions and changes were made possible because the clinics stayed open in the first place, and that was for one very simple reason: clinic staff, defenders, and escorts fought to keep them that way. For years, clinics had been left to languish by the federal government and law enforcement. Providers were harassed, stalked, and even kidnapped. Patients were unable to get inside for their appointments, unable to make their way past increasingly hostile and aggressive groups of protesters. For many years, the only thing that kept those doors open and access available were clinic escorts and defenders. They showed up, not knowing what to expect, without a playbook or a script, and figured out on their own how to keep the clinics open. They used what they had—their arms, their legs, their bodies, their voices—to form literal human chains of support and compassion for those who needed to have a simple, legal medical procedure. They were pushed, shoved, beaten, and bruised, but they kept showing up to support patients and to show the community that abortion was something worth supporting, that people who had abortions were worth supporting.

"We made the woman visible in the issue," said Jeanne Clark, a veteran clinic escort and defender from the 1980s. "The antiabortion forces' main goal was to have abortions done on invisible women with visible fetuses. We gave visibility to women. We gave that control to women. We gave that visual route and I saw it firsthand, how the majority of people, women and men, became more and more accepting."[106]

For years in Fort Wayne, women would come up to Ann Horn in the grocery store or around town to thank her for helping them "back then." It always reminded her why she did what she did: "I feel like every time I was there—I got confirmation over the years from many of them—frankly, if I made a difference to one patient or the person who was driving them, then it was worth it."[107]

If the start of 1993 marked a new feeling of momentum and success for clinic escorts and defenders, the end of 1993 would look very different. While blockades were fading into the background, another much more frightening tactic was on its way.

Two

I Fought the Law and the Law Won

DANDY BARRETT WAS ENJOYING A WARM, LEISURELY SHOWER in her Connecticut home on the morning of July 29, 1994, when the phone rang. She threw on a robe and walked over to her nightstand to answer it, dripping water along the way. It was her brother, Bruce, calling long distance from Pensacola, Florida. "Hey buddy, how are you?" she asked warmly.

Bruce was in tears, struggling to keep composure in his voice. "Dad's been shot at the Ladies Center," he said quietly. "He's dead, Dandy."[1]

• • •

To James Barrett, a life well lived meant a life lived in the service of others. He spent twenty-eight years in the air force, flying fighter planes in World War II, Korea, and Vietnam. Since retiring from the military in 1969, Barrett continued that commitment to service, first as a junior high school math and science teacher, then as a committed community volunteer.[2] When he and his wife June moved to Pensacola in 1992, seventy-two-year-old Barrett wasted no time forming a community block watch and greeting every new family with a "Welcome to the neighborhood!" He drove voters to the polls and manned the Earth Day table at the county fair. Known for his gregarious and vivacious demeanor, a quick trip to the grocery store would become a two-hour affair because he just couldn't stop talking to his neighbors. He loved to support and serve others, and he was beloved by his community in return.

In March 1993, his Pensacola community was rocked when Michael Griffin, an antiabortion protester, shot and killed Dr. David Gunn outside Pensacola Women's Health Services.[3] It was the first murder of an abortion provider in American history.

At the time, James Barrett had never been particularly politically active, but the murder of Dr. Gunn horrified and outraged him and June. Pressed by her to take action, they began to look for a way to get involved and learned that Dr. John Bayard Britton, who had replaced Dr. Gunn after his assassination, was now also facing serious harassment. Dr. Britton, one of only a few physicians left who continued to provide abortions in Pensacola, would fly in regularly from his hometown of Jacksonville, more than 350 miles away. Guaranteeing his safety was of paramount importance to the Ladies Center clinic staff, where he provided abortion care, and to the Pensacola community that Barrett loved so much.

James and June Barrett decided to help ensure that Dr. Britton could get to the clinic safely. They decided to become clinic escorts.

When he called Dandy to tell her about his new volunteer activity, she simultaneously beamed with pride and feared for his safety. But she knew that her father wasn't one to shy away from standing up for what's right. "I was proud as punch," she told me. Right before she hung up the phone, she said, "Keep your buttons shaved," an old army phrase her father often used.[4] It referenced the days of trench warfare, when soldiers would have to keep as close to the ground as possible to stay safe—so close, their buttons "shaved" the ground.

He was well aware of the risks. It didn't matter. Volunteering as a clinic escort was something worth doing, and he was going to do it. "I've spent my life doing my best for the security of my country and the people who live in it," Barrett told a local newspaper about his new volunteer activity. "Why should I stop now?"[5]

For sixteen months, James and June Barrett poured themselves into escorting. The fourth Friday of every month, they picked up Dr. Britton at the airport and drove him to the clinic. They watched as the number of protesters continued to increase. Some quietly stood and held vigil, praying to themselves. Others, like thirty-year-old Paul Hill, were more aggressive, shouting "Mommy, Mommy, don't kill me" at women approaching the clinic, and "Murderer!" at Dr. Britton. At times, they even tried to physically block him and patients from entering the clinic at all. The Barretts became adept at navigating the chaos, always staying calm under pressure, to ensure that Dr. Britton and patients got safely inside.

The air was surprisingly cool on the morning of July 29, 1994, when the Barretts drove their truck to the Pensacola Regional Airport to pick up Dr. Britton.[6] Traffic was light as they made their way back to the clinic, pulling into the parking lot just before 7:30 a.m. As the Barretts prepared to step outside and escort Dr. Britton from the car, Paul Hill calmly walked up and began firing his 12-gauge shotgun directly into the truck. James Barrett and Dr. Britton, who was wearing a bulletproof vest, were both shot in the head and killed. June Barrett was hit by bullet shrapnel in the arm and the breast but survived to tell the horrible tale of her husband's murder before her own eyes.

That day, James Barrett made history: he became the first clinic escort to die in the line of duty.

• • •

Dandy Barrett listened breathlessly as her brother recounted the call he had received from his friend Chris, who just happened to be returning a movie to a video rental store across the street from the clinic moments after Paul Hill opened fire. Chris could see a body, splayed across the pavement, covered by a tarp. He couldn't identify who it was, but he knew that truck: it belonged to Bruce's dad, James.

The rest of the conversation is a blur lost to trauma and time for Dandy. Somehow, after the truth sank in, she booked a flight to Pensacola to handle the aftermath of her father's murder.

• • •

By the time Dandy Barrett's flight touched down, Pensacola had become infamous for antiabortion assassinations. Her father had decided to become a clinic escort specifically *because* of the murder of Dr. David Gunn in March 1993. His slaying sent shock waves across the United States, signaling a new era in terrorism against abortion providers.

But it wasn't a surprise to the thousands of clinic escorts and defenders. For nearly two decades, they had seen firsthand the antiabortion movement escalate both its words and its actions. The early, co-opted language of nonviolence and civil rights traditions fell by the wayside, replaced by language like Randall Terry's rallying cry: "If you think abortion is murder, then act like it's murder."[7]

In 1992, WANTED posters had appeared around Pensacola with Dr. Gunn's face on them, along with his schedule and estimated time of arrival and departure at every clinic where he provided abortions across the Southeast.[8] Testifying before a congressional committee three weeks after his father's murder, David Gunn Jr. recalled the series of threats he had received in the weeks leading up to his murder, both over the phone and in person. Local law enforcement had merely shrugged. "They did nothing," he told Congress. "They didn't offer any help. They said, 'That's not our problem.'"

After so many years with no support from the federal government—time and again, the Justice Department under presidents Ronald Reagan and George H. W. Bush refused to use any legal tools at all to protect clinics and patients that were under increasing siege[9]—Dr. Gunn's assassination was the inevitable point to which that unchecked aggression had been leading. Finally, after his murder, with a Democrat in the White House and both the House and the Senate under Democratic control, Congress was ready to act.

Time to Face the Music

Anne Griffin (last name changed for privacy) was enjoying breakfast at a diner in Falls Church, Virginia, in 1985 when she heard a ruckus outside. She glanced up from her plate and saw a group of people swarming around a woman walking toward the front door of an abortion clinic. The group was yelling and thrusting papers in the woman's face until she made it inside. *This is disgusting*, Griffin thought. But she didn't do anything about it until four years later.

In 1989, she went to a meeting of a new coalition called the Washington Area Clinic Defense Task Force (WACDTF) and decided to become a clinic escort. Something about the simple, straightforward nature of the role appealed to her. "All I needed to do was show up," she said. "Just by showing up, I was doing enough."

WACDTF was a stabilizing force, mobilizing newly energized volunteers to take action and defend the clinics in a way that helped patients and established some semblance of structure. "Initially, we'd go stand there and link arms, and that was effective," Griffin remembered. "But when things started to get a bit more confrontational, there wasn't any protocol in place. With WACDTF and the establishment of protocols and guidelines, at least from my perspective as an escort, it made things a little less chaotic."[10]

By 1992, WACDTF was a well-oiled machine of integrated clinic defense and clinic escorting. Defenders would head to a clinic as early as 2:00 a.m. to protect against a blockade and report to WACDTF headquarters. If a blockade was in progress, defenders and escorts worked together, with defenders forming a human chain to block the protesters while escorts maneuvered around them to walk patients into the clinic.

WACDTF took its responsibility seriously, not just as a group of escorts and defenders, but as a voice for what was really happening at clinics. In May 1992, the organization testified before the House Subcommittee on Crime and Criminal Justice. A colorful cast of characters, overseen by Chairman Chuck Schumer, filled the room, from Sylvia Doe, the woman who was traumatized trying to access an abortion during the Summer of Mercy, to Randall Terry and Joseph Scheidler.[11] Tucked in at the very end of the three-and-a-half-hour hearing was a prepared statement from WACDTF, on behalf of its more than three thousand members, that spelled out exactly where clinic escorts and defenders stood. It cited several attempts by Operation Rescue to blockade clinics, the lengths to which WACDTF volunteers had to go to try to keep clinics open, and law enforcement's lack of willingness to take it seriously.

WACDTF included some of its most dramatic encounters with Operation Rescue, including an instance in January 1992. "Escorts were taking a patient through the line blockaders when one Operation Rescue member broke from the crowd, launched himself into the air and flung his body headlong into the patient and her protectors, knocking them to the ground. Although the patient attempted to press assault charges, the man was charged simply with 'incommoding,' fined $25, and set free immediately."[12]

The statement made clear why existing legal remedies weren't enough to protect clinics: "The prospect of penalties no more significant than a parking ticket enables Operation Rescue to recruit literally hundreds of people to break the law over and over again. They are able to return to break the law over and over because almost without exception, all those arrested are released within hours. This 'revolving door' system leads to massive costs for already-overburdened local law enforcement."

Left with no support from the federal government, individual clinics and local municipalities were essentially forced to play whack-a-mole with Operation Rescue. While Buffalo managed to obtain an injunction that would bar Operation Rescue from getting within fifteen feet of the clinics, protesters still willingly violated it. And Buffalo's injunction did nothing to protect clinics in other cities and states. In Milwaukee in 1992, clinics were able to obtain a temporary injunction that barred allies of Operation Rescue from getting within twenty-five feet of the city's clinics, but that only applied to Milwaukee County for a certain period of time, and it only applied to that one group.[13] It did nothing to protect clinics to the west in Madison or across the border in Chicago.

Since its inception, Operation Rescue had preyed upon this system, knowing its rank and file faced few if any consequences for willfully trespassing on clinic property during protests in Los Angeles, Milwaukee, Wichita, Buffalo, and elsewhere. Sometimes, as in Wichita, the Operation Rescue protesters would be removed by police, driven away in a bus, only to return to the clinic in a matter of hours.[14] The law wasn't stopping them; clinic escorts and defenders were.

"A federal law is urgently needed to counter the efforts of a national organization that is delighted to use our legal system against itself," WACDTF's statement concluded. "Operation Rescue leaders brag to their followers that they are 'above the law'; we need the U.S. Congress to prove that they are not."

That hearing was nearly a year before Dr. Gunn was murdered; with a Republican in the White House, Democrats in Congress weren't willing to push for legislation that might be vetoed. By 1993, the president had changed. With Dr. Gunn's murder, so had the stakes. Senator Ted Kennedy introduced the Freedom of Access to Clinic Entrances (FACE) Act on March 23, 1993, just two weeks after Dr. Gunn's murder.[15] The bill imposed severe fines and possible prison terms for both violent and nonviolent offenders—and, for the first time, provided clear federal protection to patients seeking to enter an abortion clinic.

After a year of back-and-forth hearings, Congress passed the FACE Act in the spring of 1994 with broad bipartisan support; more than two-thirds of the Senate voted in favor, including eighteen Republicans.[16] On May 26, 1994, President Bill Clinton signed it into law in front of an audience of supporters, including clinic defenders such as Ellie Smeal of the Feminist Majority Foundation, and the son and daughter of the late Dr. David Gunn.[17]

For years, clinic staff and escorts had been begging the federal government to intervene, to take the harassment and violence they were experiencing seriously, to protect the rights of patients and staff, to do *something*. Now they had a federal law, and they were ready to use it.

But while the FACE Act made clinic defense unnecessary, it didn't have the same effect on clinic escorting. Abortion opponents weren't going to stop protesting; they were just going to find new ways to do it.

• • •

Anne Griffin clutched a raggedy piece of paper against her bright orange vest near Washington, D.C.'s Maryland border. She walked the perimeter of the entrance of the abortion clinic where she had volunteered for five years, back and forth, watching for patients, monitoring the protesters.

Griffin's clinic, a walk-up that was right on a public sidewalk, faced some of the most brutal tactics from sidewalk counselors and Operation Rescue during the late 1980s and early '90s. "It was total chaos," she told me.

But the atmosphere at Griffin's clinic changed. By the fall of 1994, Griffin and her cohorts were noticing that the massive blockades had largely stopped. Operation Rescue members were no longer chaining themselves to the front door of the clinic.

In Griffin's hand was the main reason why: a copy of the newly enacted FACE Act.

While certain clinics had specific injunctions and restrictions before 1994, the FACE Act finally made it a federal crime to blockade a clinic. Clinics in every single city and every single state had a federal law that protected their entrances, and while it didn't specify how close protesters could be to the entrance, it was clear that they couldn't block it or even threaten to block it. That was now a felony. They would face serious penalties if they tried it.

Along with years of successful clinic defense, the stiff penalties in the FACE Act helped deter Operation Rescue and other antiabortion fanatics from the most serious violations. "There was less of that physical confrontation blockading, less of the locks being glued, and that kind of stuff," Griffin remembered. "My sense is that it did make a difference."

By 1994, Claire Keyes's Allegheny Reproductive Health Center in Pittsburgh, Pennsylvania, had spent a decade facing some of the most extreme antiabortion protests in the country. In 1989, it was a site of a brutal early-morning "lock-and-block" in which four men and a seventeen-year-old boy chained themselves to the underside of a car parked in front of her clinic. Keyes watched in horror as they remained there for hours, until authorities finally used a power saw to "cut through the steel locks and bars, and firefighters had to use a pumper hose and water-soaked towels to protect the demonstrators from flying sparks."[18] The Sunday of Memorial Day weekend in 1990, Keyes had to respond to another disaster: the clinic had been firebombed. No one was investigated for the crime.[19]

A year later, Laura Horowitz, a newly minted clinic escort and mother of two who was recovering from breast cancer, came face-to-face with the chaotic power of antiabortion protesters at Keyes's clinic. "They would get four hundred to five hundred people every weekend, lining the sidewalks, making it virtually impossible for anybody to get by without going through what was essentially a gauntlet of people screaming and holding up those horrible, gory signs," she said. "And screaming at them about how they were murderers and whores and sluts and killing their babies and they were going to Hell. At that time, they liked to fulminate about how clinics were giving people AIDS."[20]

Clinic escorts like Laura Horowitz were the only reason that patients were still able to get inside the clinic at all, until the FACE Act.

"Pre-FACE Act, the antis were able to stand right up into the doorway of the clinic," Horowitz said. "You would walk patients through this gauntlet on the sidewalk with literature being shoved at you and signs being shoved at your face and you'd get up to the door of the clinic and they'd be in the doorway, blocking the door." But once it became law, the atmosphere outside the clinic changed quickly. "We were overjoyed," Horowitz remembered.[21]

The blockades largely stopped. Protesters were still there, but the mass of bodies was gone. Abortion opponents were wary of outright blocking the door, unsure of how this new federal law would be implemented and what kinds of serious, punitive charges they would have to face.

Keyes finally had a moment to breathe. "After the years of siege, that is really when my life as a clinic director could be ever more focused on our mission, the women that we were there to serve," Keyes recalled. "Because I never had to pay any attention to the street, so I could be with patients. I could be with staff. I could be out in the waiting room, talking to support persons. I could be doing what it was that I loved doing."[22]

Massive protests were still taking place at many clinics, including in big cities like Boston and Chicago, but the protesters weren't blocking the entrance of the clinics anymore. "FACE made a lot of difference," said Julie Magidson, a clinic escort in Milwaukee since 1990. "They couldn't just go sit in front of the door and get slapped on the wrist and let go for the next day. That made a lot of difference."[23]

In 1995, the Feminist Majority Foundation's annual clinic violence survey found that, for the first time in the survey's three-year history, violent incidents at clinics had actually decreased.[24] They credited the FACE Act with spurring that first-of-its-kind decline.

A 1998 report to Congress on the efficacy of the FACE Act revealed what clinic escorts in WACDTF and Pittsburgh had seen firsthand: there was a dramatic reduction in clinic blockades. Nearly two in three clinics reported blockades from 1992 to 1994, but only 14 percent of clinics reported blockades from 1996 to 1998.[25] Clinics also reported a significant reduction in vandalism, bomb and arson threats, and invasions. Overall, clinics agreed that since the FACE Act's passage, there was a pronounced change in both the frequency and severity of antiabortion hostility.[26]

Susan Frietsche, a lawyer with the Women's Law Project who

has helped bring civil FACE cases against protesters at the Allegheny Reproductive Health Center and other Pennsylvania clinics, noted that "[while] FACE doesn't cover all behavior, it covers a subset of some of the worst behavior. It covers use of force, threats of force and obstruction, and those are three really serious things that we have to protect providers against."[27] FACE didn't end harassment or protesting, but it did mitigate some of the worst aspects of it. That, in and of itself, was a victory for many providers, staff, and escorts.

Clinic defense began to seem outdated and unnecessary. In the Bay Area, BACAOR changed their name from "Bay Area Coalition Against Operation Rescue" to "Bay Area Coalition for Reproductive Rights." Buffalo United for Choice, the grassroots powerhouse that had beaten back Operation Rescue in Buffalo just two years prior, faded into the wind. In Washington, D.C., WACDTF remained and kept their name, but slowly retreated from clinic defense as a tactic, embracing clinic escorting and nonengagement with antiabortion protesters.[28]

WACDTF's shift was reflected in other groups and at clinics around the country. Physically jostling for space with protesters simply wasn't necessary anymore, and volunteers realized that their role was less about protecting the door than protecting the patients individually. The best way to do that actually required an opposite perspective from clinic defense; rather than focus on what the protesters were doing, clinic escorts needed to zero in on the patients. In Brookline, Massachusetts, the Brookline Clinic Access Team began reworking their guides, language, and tactics to reflect the shift: "The clinic escort is there to make the experience of getting in the clinic a less traumatic one for the patient. Our focus is on the patient, not the antis—we are not there to confront the antis."[29]

There seemed to be little need for clinic defense if the federal government was willing to defend the clinics instead. As the most disruptive tactics began to wane at clinics, it seemed possible that the FACE Act would do the heavy lifting, and might even make clinic escorting eventually unnecessary as well.

How Far Is Not Far Enough?

The FACE Act was passed to stop mass blockades and address burgeoning antiabortion violence, and it largely did that. But for most clinics, mass blockades and violence were not their primary problems. When Dr. Britton and James Barrett were murdered, only a handful of clinics had experienced shootings, and only one had experienced deadly shootings. Some clinics had a violence problem, but nearly every clinic had a harassment problem.

Clinic staff and escorts hoped that the FACE Act would be their opportunity to stop predatory "sidewalk counseling" and end the intrusive and persistent harassment that patients had to face just to get in the door. Clinic escort teams familiarized themselves with every detail of the FACE Act as quickly as they could, believing that if they could document what was happening, law enforcement would be ready and able to take action. WACDTF held trainings for their members on what the legislation allowed, what it prohibited, and how best to deploy it.[30]

Griffin and other WACDTF members carried their copy of the legislation with them during every shift, continually referring back to it to see if what a protester was doing would qualify as a FACE violation. Sometimes it did; a lot of the time, they just weren't sure.

It was clear that the FACE Act made the atmosphere at abortion clinics better. Unfortunately, that still didn't make it good.

In Washington, D.C., WACDTF continued their early morning "clinic watches" even after FACE was passed. "We'd try to be preventive and have teams of people in a car at a clinic or driving between clinics, starting at three in the morning," Alicia Lucksted said of WACDTF. It wasn't always successful. While the FACE Act had rendered clinic defense unnecessary, some abortion opponents were still more than willing to break the law. D.C.-area clinics still experienced "lock-and-blocks" and glued locks to such a frequent extent that Lucksted had a locksmith on speed dial.[31]

"The FACE Act didn't go all that far," said Anne Griffin. "So, we'd also know what they were still allowed to do, which was yell and scream at patients and try to stick literature in patients' hands."[32] Griffin's copy of the FACE Act became tattered, but not from actual use. Instead, she would jam it into her pocket so she could spread out her arms in a wide T to form a human buffer around a patient.

In reality, the FACE Act did little to curb protesting. The 1998 congressional report on the FACE Act's efficacy found that while the numbers of violent incidents and blockades had dramatically declined, more clinics reported picketing *after* FACE became law than before—every single clinic that responded to the survey reported picketing.[33]

• • •

"Hi, Leanne. Two more for you."

On the frigid morning of December 17, 1994, Jonathan McDowell gently nudged two patients toward Preterm Health Services staff member Leanne Nichols in Brookline, Massachusetts. Shy but kind, Nichols would check the patients in and often stop to share a few words with the escorts. McDowell smiled and waved as he headed back out into the mass of antiabortion protesters gathered out front.

Brookline, an upscale neighbor of Boston, was home to several abortion clinics. It had seen its share of blockades, and while those had ended, sizable protests remained the norm at Preterm and other

Brookline clinics. Today was no different. At least a couple hundred abortion opponents gathered out front of the clinic, holding a huge banner depicting the Virgin Mary and other signs featuring bloody and gory imagery.

McDowell, a recent immigrant from England who was pursuing a PhD in astrophysics at Harvard, was used to spotting patterns and maintaining a kind of hyperawareness. He learned to watch for irregular and unusual protesters, those who were quiet and away from the group. While the hubbub was taking place outside the clinic's front door, McDowell turned his attention to the back entrance, where only a couple of gadfly protesters were attempting to intercept patients. He saw someone new, standing by himself, just staring at the clinic.

"He had these really dead eyes," McDowell said. "He was a youngish guy and I remember commenting to the security guard, 'Keep an eye on that guy. He creeps me out.' But I didn't think any more of it. He was definitely creepy, even by the standards of Operation Rescue."[34]

McDowell felt uneasy about the new protester, but decided not to call the police. What would he report? There's a man at the clinic and he's kind of weird? The FACE Act didn't say anything about suspect behavior, only blatant intimidation and attempts to block a clinic entrance. The police had already expressed annoyance about having to protect the clinic from flagrant FACE violations; McDowell didn't want to risk annoying them further.

Thirteen days later, McDowell was in the Harvard library, trying to get some work done, when he overheard the librarian say something about a shooting at a women's health clinic. McDowell dropped his books, ran to his car, and raced to Preterm. "I saw the police tape outside, and all the TV trucks and everything."[35]

It was the second shooting at an abortion clinic in Brookline that day. Before calmly heading over to Preterm, opening the front door, and firing at will, twenty-three-year-old John Salvi, a radical antiabortion terrorist, had opened fire at Planned Parenthood League of Massachusetts. By the end of the day, Salvi had shot five people, and two were dead: PPLM's twenty-five-year-old receptionist Shannon Lowney, and Leanne Nichols, McDowell's friend at Preterm.[36]

McDowell knew both women, though he was closer to Nichols. Lost in the glare of bright yellow police tape, he thought back to the creepy man he had seen a couple weeks earlier behind the building that was now a harrowing crime scene. "I think that was John Salvi," he muttered to himself. His stomach churned. He recalled his conversation with the security guard, Richard J. Sarone, who chased Salvi after he opened fire at Preterm. He remembered deciding not to call the police, fearing they wouldn't take him seriously.

The next morning, Saturday, December 31, Salvi was still on the loose. Preterm and PPLM were closed, both still active crime scenes. But the staff at the other abortion clinic in Brookline, Reproductive Health Associates, decided to keep the clinic open that day. McDowell and the other members of the Brookline Clinic Access Team decided that they too would show up. They gathered out front, put on their neon vests, and stood in the bitter cold for hours, standing guard, opening the door for terrified patients, diligently watching every protester who showed up.

McDowell spotted Bill Carter, a local Operation Rescue protester he knew. "You really want to be here today?" McDowell asked him. "What about the people who died?"

"What about the babies inside the clinic who are dying today?" Carter responded.[37]

McDowell said nothing. He just shook his head and went back to standing guard. He wasn't there for Carter. He was there for the patients. He was there to memorialize Lowney and Nichols. He was there to try to prevent another tragedy like this from happening again.

Salvi was arrested less than a week later after shooting up an abortion clinic in Norfolk, Virginia. Mercifully, no one was injured.

By the end of 1994, five abortion providers and clinic staff, including a clinic escort, had been murdered by antiabortion terrorists. The limits of the FACE Act were on full display, and clinic escorts were, once again, the first and last line of defense.

• • •

Leslie Fillingham had seen the lengths to which protesters would go to block access to a clinic, and she had the bruises to prove it. While on the clinic defense line in Milwaukee during an Operation Rescue blockade in 1992, "I can remember being in front of the clinic and this group just sort of charging us. I got knocked into a wall and bruised my ribs." When the FACE Act became law, Fillingham was filled with hope. "I distinctly remember the FACE Act being passed. I have a necklace [in its honor] that one of our members made," she remembered. She wore it, tucked under her clinic escort vest, every time she showed up for a shift at her clinic.[38]

Her hope turned out to be in vain. Milwaukee did manage to obtain an injunction that kept blockaders twenty-five feet away from the clinic before the FACE Act, but that was temporary. They always came back.

The FACE Act prohibited blocking or attempting to block entrance to a clinic, but it didn't specify how far away from the clinic the protesters had to be. They simply couldn't block the entrance. But was standing by the door and leaning into a patient as she walked in "blocking" the entrance? What about walking in front of a patient the entire walk to the front door?

Milwaukee police didn't know, and even if they did arrest someone, they didn't get to decide whether charges would be brought.

"The problem in Milwaukee was that a lot of this activity even
before FACE was illegal; however the [district attorney] in Milwaukee at the time was a devout Catholic," Fillingham said. "He had a
blind spot about the antis. The police would arrest them for disorderly conduct and the DA would let them go."

The FACE Act empowered the Justice Department to bring
criminal charges against those who violated the law, but that required the political will to do so. In places like Milwaukee and Pittsburgh, cities with large Catholic populations, aversion to abortion
was common among those in positions of power. While clinics could
try to bring civil FACE cases against violators, that required a significant amount of time and money, something most clinics didn't
have. And even if they did win that case, it wouldn't bring a criminal
penalty, just a financial one.

• • •

Clinic escorts also took on the ambitious task of documenting FACE
violations for apathetic law enforcement, trying mightily to give the
legislation the teeth it needed to protect the patients they served.
From the beginning, WACDTF leaders realized that while the
FACE Act gave law enforcement the power to intervene in cases of
blockades, it would be up to escorts and staff to flag a FACE violation
in the first place.

Unfortunately, the existence of the FACE Act didn't translate
into widespread education for law enforcement on what it was or
how to enforce it. In many cities, including Washington, D.C., police were still wary of intervening, and since the massive blockades
had largely stopped, many officers and city officials thought that the

problem had been solved for them. But FACE didn't stop protesters from getting in the faces of patients. It didn't stop them from screaming "Murderer! Jezebel!" at every woman who walked by the clinic. It didn't impose restrictions on the noise level, or stop the protesters from filming the faces and license plates of clinic staff and abortion patients.

Law enforcement either didn't want to deal with that, or didn't feel that FACE gave them the ability to do it.

While the FACE Act freed up Claire Keyes to dedicate more of her energy to her patients, her clinic escorts now added "monitoring and documenting potential felonies" to their to-do list. "To have reliable people who, post-FACE, could recognize what a FACE violation was and what wasn't; there are people who can do a part of what [our escorts] did but there aren't very many who can do all of what they do," Keyes said. "And that really made a difference."[39]

Laura Horowitz and the rest of her team began to more formally record every shift outside the clinic and share information with each other. Her team in Pittsburgh developed the new role of "coordinator," who would serve as the lead for a given shift and lead on interactions with both clinic staff and law enforcement, if necessary, something Claire Keyes believed helped immeasurably.

"They were the ones who developed a really good relationship with the police, because the police didn't want to be called every fifteen minutes that some protester had broken the law. So, they were very judicious when they would have to involve the police. The police came to trust and respect what it was that they were doing. I can't say enough good about them. They were just unbelievable, and they're still there."[40]

But while the relationship with law enforcement improved, it didn't change the efficacy of the FACE Act. The Pittsburgh clinic escort coordinators were tasked with writing a formal report covering what happened every week at the clinic. "Once we had FACE, we could say, 'This was blocking under FACE, this would be harassment, this would be stalking,' so we'd put that in."[41] Every week, the coordinator would write and file the formal report, and every week, nothing would happen. "We never had a FACE Act violation filed here, despite the fact that providers have been harassed at home, followed on the street, doors have been blockaded, clinics have been damaged.[42]

"I think we felt that the FACE Act was going to be great, that it was going to get the demonstrators away from the patients and give us a valuable legal tool," Horowitz said. "This is just not something that happens, FACE prosecutions by the [federal authorities]. It feels like a betrayal. It was not easy to get FACE passed, and not following through with it, it just adds insult to injury."[43]

As of 1998, one in four clinics that experienced picketing from abortion opponents reported that they weren't satisfied with law enforcement's response, precisely because of what was happening to Horowitz and other Pittsburgh clinic defenders.[44] Ultimately, they were often left to their own devices, knowing that law enforcement was reluctant or even unwilling to come out and deal with an isolated incident of individualized harassment. In many ways, Horowitz and others had to attempt to enforce the law on their own, trying to wield the threat of the FACE Act against unruly protesters who crossed the line but not badly enough for a police officer to come down to the clinic.

Ann Horn was facing the same situation in Fort Wayne, Indiana. After years battling with Joseph Scheidler, Operation Rescue, and other antiabortion protesters, Horn was an old hand at clinic escorting. She knew that the Fort Wayne Police Department simply wasn't interested in policing the clinic or dealing with the antics of the protesters, so Horn took it upon herself.

"With the regular protesters, it was different [after the FACE Act]. But I knew the people, and I could tell by their behavior. A lot of times, you really could prevent things . . . There were certain really scary characters and when they came around, I would not let [the clinic staff] release patients. I'd just say, 'Don't release anybody now, staff don't come outside to smoke.' And I'd keep my eye on him. [One male protester] tried to get in once and I just leaned hard against that door. I got so you could tell from their behavior. They're fairly predictable. If you watch their behavior, you can tell. It's like, okay, something could happen. If you saw it in time, you could usually keep it from being too big an issue."[45]

Horn became so adept at securing the Fort Wayne clinic that by the end of the 1990s, she traded her neon vest for a badge—she became the clinic's full-time security guard.

Protesting's Face-Lift

In terms of access, FACE helped remove one roadblock. But the process of a patient trying to access an abortion remained an obstacle course. While there might not be hundreds of people screaming into a patient's car window anymore, there were still dozens of people in her face, screaming, shoving things at her, trying to grab her, walking directly in front of her.

Melina Gesell was a twenty-one-year-old student at Barnard College in New York City in 1995 when she spoke to *The New York Times* about her experience as a clinic escort in the city. Protesters found ways to hinder access without overtly blocking the entrance. "In addition to the verbal harassment, the anti-choice protesters had little pamphlets depicting alleged, supposed fetuses. They would thrust them in the patients' faces, try to throw them into the windows of cars. Then there was the physical harassment. They were permitted to physically intercept and stand directly in front of people, and walk backwards in an attempt to block patients from entering."[46]

Clinic escorts weren't the only ones who studied the FACE Act; the protesters did too, and they quickly learned how far they could push without consequence. Protesters soon reverted to the tactics of their original star, Joseph Scheidler. In the early 1980s, Scheidler's *Closed: 99 Ways to Stop Abortion* formalized the haphazard harassment and protesting tactics that would become a permanent fixture in a post-FACE America. Scheidler's book helped legitimize "sidewalk counseling," a term that belies the cruelty of the practice. Abortion opponents claim that sidewalk counseling is meant to simply provide abortion patients with information and another option, as if abortion patients aren't informed and haven't already made the best decision for themselves. "Sidewalk counselors" get right in patients' faces, often before they even emerge from their car or the subway, and begin peppering them with horrific language and gruesome photos. Scheidler's *Closed* made clear that protesters should use deliberately "inflammatory language" when talking to patients.

"Are you going into the abortion chamber?"[47]

"Your baby has a heart!"

"Women who reject God's gift, his children, he makes them barren. Because women become sterile out of abortion."[48]

"How does it feel to be the mother of a dead baby?"

"Before God, you have now become a murderer!"[49]

Scheidler's recommendations for sidewalk counselors took on a new life after the FACE Act. Protesters could no longer block the clinic's doors. Instead, they tried to take up residence inside the minds of abortion patients, and clinic escorts would have to try to keep them out.

• • •

Shanna Atchley-Shafer was fresh out of high school in 1996 the first time she ever visited an abortion clinic. The procedure wasn't for her—a pregnant family member had asked Atchley-Shafer to be her support person, and she accepted.

"[My family member] was a little nervous going," Atchley-Shafer said, remembering their car ride to Planned Parenthood in Omaha, Nebraska. "[There was] a lot of joking and camaraderie in the car to diffuse any sort of nervousness on her side. She was also very confident in her decision, and we supported her wholeheartedly."

They parked the car and Atchley-Shafer and another friend of the patient helped her out of the car. They could hear shouting—"You're a baby killer!" "You don't have to be the mother of a dead baby!" Her family member grabbed Atchley-Shafer's hand, exhaling sharply, preparing to walk through the impending gauntlet. That's when Atchley-Shafer noticed three women in bright neon vests walking swiftly toward them. This clinic had escorts.

The vested women began to walk with the group toward the clinic's front steps. One middle-aged woman spoke in a calm, gentle tone, encouraging the group to listen to her, not to anyone else. Her voice was almost hypnotic; its softness helped Atchley-Shafer and the others to focus on her, rather than the horrific insults that were being hurled at them.

Atchley-Shafer could almost feel the rage vibrating from the protesters who had swarmed around the group. "They were very close," she remembered. The trio of clinic escorts was the only barrier between the protesters' angry screams and gory fetus pictures and the patient and her supporters.

The clinic escorts walked past the mob, through the gate, and up the steps. Atchley-Shafer heard a protester shout at her loved one, "Think of all the people who want babies and can't have them!" She turned her head sharply, just in time to see one of their clinic escorts shut the protester down and physically cut off his access to the group. After her loved one and friend entered the clinic, Atchley-Shafer stood at the door, in awe of these women and what they had just done.

"I was like, Wow, this is awesome . . . At that point, all I'd experienced was pro-life/pro-choice. It was very black and white. I just remember being so grateful to have someone that was able to verbalize anything beyond that basic black and white. It was actually a pretty formative day for me."

Atchley-Shafer stayed outside to chat with the clinic escorts, inquiring about how long they'd been doing this, what it was like, how they kept their cool. She marveled at how they managed to stay calm, how they never asked personal questions of the patients or their companions but rather offered calm, reassuring, vague statements of support. They explained that the protesters had been coming for a long time but had been screaming even louder lately, since they couldn't block the entrance anymore.

When Atchley-Shafer needed an abortion nearly two decades later, there were no clinic escorts. But she remembered how strong they were that day, replaying their gentle tone in her head as she walked through the mass of protesters by herself.[50]

• • •

Benita Ulisano began volunteering as a clinic escort and defender in the early 1990s in Chicago, and she quickly became accustomed to large crowds and a persistent tension in the air. The FACE Act didn't change that for her.

"Even though the FACE Act had been enacted, [antiabortion groups] would just bring out larger groups, lots and lots—hundreds, at certain times—larger groups, from our perspective," Ulisano told

me. "It was just so different, closer proximity . . . It just seemed a
lot more aggressive in a different way, a more physical, in-your-face
way."[51]

That "in-your-face" aspect of protesting made it as uncomfortable and painful for a person seeking an abortion as possible. And
because FACE was narrowly focused on prohibiting protesters from
blocking the entrance to a clinic, it gave them unchecked license to
target individuals entering the clinic for focused harassment. As a result, clinic escorts' role became less about physically battling to keep
a clinic open than using their bodies as a source of individualized
support. The protesters' targets weren't clinic entrances anymore;
they were patients trying to get in the door.

"One of the goals of escorting a patient is to make sure that
they are listening to you and not to what's being screamed at them,"
Laura Horowitz of Pittsburgh said. Rather than forming massive
human chains around a patient, Horowitz and others would gently
approach them farther away from the clinic and develop a personal
connection, calmly explaining what was happening and who they
were. "We [developed] this kind of script that we use that's pretty
content-free, but it's intended to give them something to listen to
on the way up the street. We're careful not to say or ask anything
personal . . . we just walk with them."

Clinic escorting became a role focused primarily on serving the
individualized needs of the patient. This was more or less impossible
during the years of blockades—with hundreds of protesters trying
to block the clinic, a clinic escort would simply walk the patient
through a narrow pathway created by the clinic defense team. It
wasn't about meeting that patient where they were or even creating a
calming environment for them. It was just about getting them in the
door as safely and quickly as possible.

The soothing, gentle tones that guided Shanna Atchley-Shafer and her family member through the mobs of protesters in Omaha in 1996 were based on this newer model of clinic escorting. Instead of loudly shouting down the protesters, escorts would get down on the individual, human level of the patients. Calming voices, simple statements, and one-on-one connections began to dominate the practice. Neither the FACE Act nor clinic escorts could stop protesters from coming to clinics. But clinic escorts could mitigate the harm as much as possible by reminding every person they walked to the clinic's doors that they were human and they weren't alone.

• • •

It was early Saturday morning once again for Ellie Dorritie on October 24, 1998. Since Buffalo United for Choice (BUFC) broke apart after successfully defending the city's clinics in 1992, she hadn't had to get up in the early morning hours to try to beat Operation Rescue to the door of a clinic. But today, she was awake before the sun. She had a lot of work to do. She had to help get the band back together.[52]

But this time, it wasn't to defend a clinic.

The night before, Dr. Barnett Slepian, an abortion provider at Buffalo Women's Services, came home from synagogue with his wife. Three of his sons settled in front of the television while he walked into the kitchen with his wife and fourth son. He had barely settled in when a bullet ripped through a back window and struck him in his chest.[53] Within an hour, he was declared dead.[54]

Dr. Slepian, who had weathered years of threats and blockades, became the seventh abortion provider or clinic staff member to be murdered in the United States. The FACE Act had been law for four years, but it didn't stop the sniper's bullet from piercing the drapes in Dr. Slepian's kitchen window.

Dorritie was devastated. She had known Dr. Slepian—his clinic had been involved in BUFC's clinic defense, and he was beloved in their community. She and hundreds of others gathered, shoulder to shoulder like they had in 1992, for a candlelight vigil outside the Slepian home.

That period of grief and fear was jolted into outrage when, capitalizing off of the national media attention on Buffalo and the issue of abortion, antiabortion leaders vowed to make Buffalo their new target for protesting in the spring of 1999. It would mark seven years since Operation Rescue had been shut down by clinic defenders. Now, in the middle of grieving the loss of one of their own, Buffalo abortion rights supporters tried to figure out what to do.

"There were a lot of people who had come to the conclusion that women would be frightened and not want to come out," Dorritie said of the internal debate. "And then there were a lot of people who felt that if there were ever any time that we should try to show our power against that kind of terrorism, it was then."

The need to protect the clinics and defend Dr. Slepian's memory won out. In the wake of his murder, Buffalo United for Choice reunited. Some former members, like Dianne Mathiowetz, had left Buffalo, but most were ready and able to once again face off with Operation Rescue's spin-off organization, Operation Save America, now led by a North Carolina minister named Philip "Flip" Benham.[55]

It was chilly and windy on April 20, 1999, without a speck of the rain that came to dominate the memory of BUFC's heroic clinic defense in 1992.[56] That wasn't all that was different this time around.

"There were much fewer clinics," Dorritie told me, highlighting a trend that extended well past Buffalo. From 1995 to 2000, abortion providers—exhausted from frequent harassment and the escalating financial costs of security for the clinic and themselves—decreased by 11 percent, a trend that would continue into the new millennium.[57]

"There were only a couple clinics left in Buffalo and there was much less of a war at the time." Operation Save America decided not just to mount a protest at Buffalo's clinics, but to protest the city's gay bars and even bookstores. "That just brought out everybody."

Once again, Dorritie locked arms with many of the same people with whom she'd locked arms seven years ago. "Human chain all over again," she remembered. And they weren't alone. This time, law enforcement worked with them, rather than around them, forming a police line between Operation Save America members and the clinic defense line.[58]

Once again, the clinic escorts and defenders dramatically outnumbered the antiabortion protesters. Their effort to disrupt the clinics was even more lackluster than seven years ago, Dorritie remembered. "The only attacks at the clinic were a bunch of people with ugly signs, maybe four or five of them, standing outside the remaining Buffalo clinic at odd times."

Just like in 1992, volunteers successfully defended the clinics and other targets of the radical antiabortion protesters. But the reunion was short-lived. "There was a lot of intimidation that came with [Slepian's] murder and a lot of grief," Dorritie recalled. "It's very hard to mix grief and anger in a climate where grief is more easily accommodated. You have to be something of a radical to overcome that. It was a difficult time."[59]

· · ·

By the end of the millennium, Buffalo United for Choice had once again disbanded, and antiabortion protests and violence seemed to fade into the media and cultural background. Without Operation Rescue capturing the media with its chaotic carnival, and after the media circus around President Bill Clinton's impeachment, the issue no longer commanded the kind of splashy coverage that it had just a few years earlier.

Alicia Lucksted remembers this as a period of transition for WACDTF, shifting from reactive response to dedicated, proactive teams. "I do remember it being like, 'How do we do this? What are we doing? Is it the right thing do?' Just trying to forge and figure out, and disagree and figure it out again—and learn from others. But also, kind of make stuff up, like we had to at the beginning."

While there certainly were dedicated escorts for specific clinics before the late 1990s, the shift in antiabortion protesting after the FACE Act made that a permanent fixture. The risk to clinics wasn't large, surprise blockades anymore but quotidian, routine harassment. For the most part, the same protesters came, week in and week out, using the same rhetoric and tactics that would skirt the FACE Act but still impede patients' access. Clinic escorting was no longer a reactive response—it was now a daily act. The risk of violence and vandalism was still there, but as the new millennium dawned, the atmosphere outside the clinics largely settled into a normalized routine of "sidewalk counselors" who harassed patients and clinic escorts who tried to protect them as much as possible. Over time, this dynamic became commonplace, slowly accepted as normal by the media and the American public.

As a result, some clinic escort teams began to scale back or even fold. Not seeing as much of a need for them anymore, many clinics thought they could handle the protesters without escorts. Cities and states began to pass buffer zones that granted clinics even more reprieve. In 2007, Massachusetts enacted a thirty-five-foot buffer zone at the state's abortion clinics, one of the strongest in the nation.[60] It would be challenged in court and eventually invalidated by the Supreme Court seven years later. But for the years that it existed, it successfully kept the protesters at bay—with the barrier that the buffer zone law provided, there was no need for clinic escorts, and the Brookline Clinic Access Team quietly folded.

Many teams remained, but some of the volunteers took time away, too. In Milwaukee, Leslie Fillingham desperately needed a break. She had been protecting the city's clinics for most of the decade, and she was burned out. "Every single Saturday morning of your life, you're out there for hours and it's stressful," she said.[61] By the time she returned to clinic escorting in the early 2000s, it was largely the same protesters, on the same days, using the same rhetoric, waving the same signs. But one thing was different: the city now had only two clinics left. Little did she know it would be a harbinger of things to come in the new millennium.

· · ·

Despite its vagueness, the FACE Act undoubtedly made a difference for abortion clinics across the country. It just wasn't enough. While FACE signified that the federal government took antiabortion harassment seriously, it didn't always look that way to those on the front lines. Law enforcement had little idea how to enforce FACE, leaving clinic escorts to complain about FACE violations in vain. It stopped blockades, but it didn't stop protesters. They learned to work around it, and the new form of protesting they found—individualized harassment—not only flourished, but came to be accepted as simply normal for abortion clinics.

The FACE Act should have been a starting point. Instead, it would signal the last time Congress passed a proactive bill in defense of abortion rights.

In Pensacola, James and June Barrett would drive their pickup truck past Paul Hill. James even tried to engage Hill on occasion, attempting to persuade him to stop harassing people.[62] Hill never budged and, reportedly enraged when President Clinton signed the FACE Act into law in May 1994, began to publicly escalate his behavior and rhetoric.[63] He called the murder of Dr. Gunn "justifiable homicide"and began to scream louder and louder outside the clinic.[64]

Ladies Center administrator Linda Taggert used the FACE Act as leverage to advocate for Hill's arrest. But Pensacola police refused to intervene, telling her they had no guidelines to arrest him under the FACE Act. "I then telephoned the ATF and was referred to the FBI. Their agent said he would 'take down the information' but could not make an arrest because he had no guidelines."[65]

Dandy Barrett once again returned to Pensacola in the fall of 1994 as Paul Hill became the first person to be charged under the FACE Act. But by then, it was too late—he had already murdered her father.

Three

Too Many to Count

CORY ELLEN HELD THE PHONE TO HER EAR. STILL THROBBING with outrage and grief from the murder of abortion provider Dr. George Tiller a couple of months earlier in May 2009, Ellen exhaled sharply into the receiver. After the third ring, a voice answered. "Thank you for calling Family Planning Associates Women's Health of Los Angeles. How may I help you?"

"Hi, I'm calling because I'm interested in volunteering as a clinic escort with you all," Ellen said.

It had been more than a decade since Ellen had last volunteered at an abortion clinic. While in college in 1997, she had volunteered as a clinic escort at a Planned Parenthood in Poughkeepsie, New York, but once she graduated and moved out west, there didn't seem to be as much of a need. But she still kept tabs on what was happening in abortion rights, and when she heard about a new mass protest group emerging, she decided the summer of 2009 was the time to return to her vest.

"I heard that you all have been targeted by some group called 40 Days for Life," Ellen explained. "I want to help."

"I'm sorry, what? What are you talking about?"

"40 Days for Life. The antiabortion protest group. They're apparently coming to your clinic to stage a big protest."

"I have no idea what that is."

Ellen quickly realized that not only had this clinic staff member never heard of 40 Days for Life, the clinic didn't even have escorts. In fact, almost none of the clinics in Los Angeles did.

"It was L.A., so I obviously assumed something existed and I'd find it," Ellen said. "But it turns out it didn't, which I couldn't believe."[1]

Los Angeles was unique in terms of abortion access. When California decriminalized abortion in 1967, allowing abortions for "therapeutic" reasons like rape, the city was at the forefront of the changing tides around abortion.[2] Los Angeles was the epicenter of an underground movement, led by Carol Downer and her compatriots, to facilitate illegal but safe abortions for those who needed abortions for other reasons.[3] When Operation Rescue threatened to turn Los Angeles into the first "abortion-free city" in 1989, a new outgrowth of NOW, the National Clinic Defense Project, helped mobilize ten thousand clinic escorts and defenders to protect the city's clinics.[4]

But when the new millennium dawned, the days of mass clinic defense mobilization were a faded memory. In 2008, the city passed a "bubble zone" ordinance that required protesters to stay at least eight feet away from patients within a hundred-foot radius of the clinic. It was designed to create an invisible and impenetrable barrier around patients in place of a literal clinic escort.[5] Without the threat of massive blockades, and as the FACE Act began to take effect, it didn't seem necessary to have clinic escorts in a city like Los Angeles anymore—or at most clinics, for that matter. If even the abortion clinic that Ellen called didn't know about the 40 Days for Life protest event, how could the general public be expected to know?

Instead of throwing up her hands, Ellen decided to go one step further: she created L.A. for Choice, the city's first coordinated clinic escort group since the early days of Operation Rescue blockades. This time, they weren't facing off against Operation Rescue; they were contending with 40 Days for Life, a new, Catholic-based anti-abortion group that brought massive protests at abortion clinics back to the forefront in America.

• • •

By the FACE Act's tenth anniversary in 2004, clinic blockades were a relic of a long-gone era. There was still haphazard vandalism and violence against abortion providers, but mercifully there had been no casualties since Dr. Bart Slepian's horrific murder six years earlier. The word "terrorism" was ubiquitous in the media, but in a post–September 11 world, it referred only to one very specific type: Islamic terrorism.

Besides, abortion opponents finally had someone in the White House who they thought could get the job done for them. President George W. Bush, who ran as a "compassionate conservative," helped to usher in a new era in institutionalizing opposition to abortion.[6] As president, he appointed two abortion opponents to the Supreme Court— Chief Justice John Roberts and Justice Samuel Alito—who would long outlive Bush's own tenure and serve as two more potentially decisive votes against legal abortion. In 2003, he championed and eventually signed the Partial-Birth Abortion Ban Act, a deceptively named bill that banned dilation and extraction, a common, safe second-trimester abortion procedure.[7] Abortion opponents learned to leverage propagandistic language—the ban didn't use medical terminology—to paint abortion as gruesome, rather than as basic medical care.[8] That ban, which was subsequently upheld by the Supreme Court in 2007 (including by both of Bush's appointees), became the nation's first federal abortion ban since abortion was legalized nationwide in 1973.[9]

For the first time since *Roe*, the anti-choice cause was making significant headway in the highest echelons of power. For years, opponents had tried to restrict abortion, pushing "parental consent" laws, which required minors to have permission from one or both parents, through state legislatures, without succeeding at their ultimate goal—overturning *Roe v. Wade*. With Bush in the White House and a Supreme Court that was no longer solidly in support of the landmark ruling, abortion opponents turned their attention to the long game. They might not be able to ban abortion right *now*, but the gains during the Bush presidency could potentially pay dividends in years to come. They didn't need to stage massive protests at abortion clinics. They could wage war from within the halls of power.

While the diehards were still standing outside the clinics, anti-abortion protesters had more or less become a pitiable anachronism in American popular consciousness and culture. The same year that the Supreme Court upheld a federal abortion ban, the comedy *Juno*, about a teenage girl who becomes pregnant and decides to give the baby up for adoption, reinforced this narrative with the character of Su-Chin, the lone teenage protester outside the one abortion clinic to which Juno goes. "All babies want to get borned!" Su-Chin sweetly chants, noticing her classmate Juno. Su-Chin tells Juno that her baby has "fingernails" before Juno decides to enter the clinic anyway.[10] This image of a sweet, well-intentioned protester, worthy of both our pity and an eye roll, became the dominant caricature of an antiabortion protester in the first decade of the new millennium.

That mythical caricature belied the emergence of a new and reenergized national antiabortion protest movement, fueled by the legislative wins to come. At the beginning of the 2000s, clinics that featured robust clinic escort teams were used to dealing with the same handful of protesters year after year. In fact, some clinics managed to avoid protesters altogether, flying under the radar as abortion opponents reveled in the anti-choice Bush administration from 2001 to 2008. As George W. Bush departed and Barack Obama took office in January 2009, many abortion clinic staff knew what to expect: an uptick in protesters.

"Protests increase when Democrats are in office," explained Amy Hagstrom Miller, CEO of Whole Woman's Health. "It's an interesting tit-for-tat. When a Democrat is in office, antiabortion people go crazy, and violence increases."[11] Hagstrom Miller would take center stage in the judicial fight against abortion restrictions in the 2010s.

The inauguration of the nation's first Black president coincided with the reemergence of massive antiabortion protests at clinics across the country. The right-wing backlash against President Obama helped trigger the beginning of the most restrictive decade for abortion rights in recent memory.

• • •

By 2005, it had been more than a decade since Benita Ulisano last donned a neon vest at an abortion clinic. The Chicago native had spent a couple of years as a clinic escort and defender in the 1990s, going back and forth to different Chicago-area clinics as needed.[12] Ulisano witnessed the effects and limitations of the FACE Act up close and personal during those years. "For whatever reason, the matriarchs of the organizations that were running the clinic escort program decided that it might be too dangerous and folded the program, thinking that if we left, they would leave," Ulisano said of the escort group's eventual disbanding at the end of the decade. "There was a time when there was no clinic escorting available because clinics weren't using us."

But by the late 2000s, Ulisano had been hearing talk of a new group that was bringing tens, sometimes hundreds of protesters to clinics during the Lent season.[13] They called themselves 40 Days for Life, the same group Cory Ellen had tried to warn Family Planning Associates about in Los Angeles in 2009.

What became 40 Days for Life began outside a Planned Parenthood in Bryan, Texas, in 2004.[14] Led by an abortion opponent named David Bereit, a local antiabortion group called the Brazos Valley Coalition for Life had decided to stage a nonstop, twenty-four-hour sit-in at the Planned Parenthood clinic. Unlike other protests, this one continued for years. As 2004 became 2005, the Planned Parenthood in Bryan became the most protested clinic in the country because of the group's daily sit-in.[15] Bereit gained national recognition when he extended the protest in Bryan to a massive community boycott against a Planned Parenthood in Austin that sought to expand its operations. By 2007, his isolated sit-in effort had become a national organization, dedicated to bringing massive numbers of protesters to abortion clinics during two six-week periods in the spring and the fall. Critical to their brand, 40 Days for Life claims that they aren't "protesting," but rather "keeping vigil" to end abortion.[16] The organization didn't block entrances like their forerunners in Operation Rescue, but simply used their sheer size, interwoven with sinister "sidewalk counseling," to intimidate patients and interfere with clinic staff's ability to do their jobs. At that point, no other antiabortion group could bring that number of people to a clinic or disrupt patient comfort at the same level as 40 Days for Life.

And now they were coming to Chicago. For Ulisano, this sounded eerily similar to what she had seen in the early 1990s, except this time, there weren't any clinic escorts. "It disturbed me that we weren't at the clinics anymore after our group dismantled in the nineties," she said.[17] She and other members of the newly formed

Illinois Choice Action Team (ICAT), a statewide arm of NARAL, contacted Chicago-area clinics that were facing 40 Days for Life protests with offers to "counterprotest." It wasn't clinic escorting—they didn't interact with patients. Instead, they attempted to distract the 40 Days protesters. If nothing else, they just wanted to show the community that there was support for the clinics.

"At first, they were like, 'No!'" Ulisano recalled of their offer to clinics. "But [clinic staff] liked us there because we were respectful." Ulisano and others remained off property, away from patients.[18] Instead, they stood to the side, holding signs that said YOUR BODY YOUR CHOICE and THIS CLINIC STAYS OPEN!

For forty days, come rain, shine, or (often during Lent) frigid cold and piles of snow, hundreds of protesters gathered at abortion clinics across Chicago. Operation Rescue had a fundamentalist and evangelical component, but 40 Days for Life was Catholic. Huge banners of the Virgin Mary would abound outside the Family Planning Associates clinic. Hundreds of people, some praying the rosary, others "sidewalk counseling" and pleading with patients to turn around and save themselves from hell, would swarm around the clinics. The pro-choice counterprotesters didn't and couldn't intercept the patients. They had to stand to the side and watch. The clinic staff were wary of allowing full-time escorts to resume, fearful it would make the situation worse.

The staff at Family Planning Associates soon realized that "worse" was already there. Because Ulisano and others were technically counterprotesters, they couldn't engage with patients. Instead, she simply watched as the numbers of protestors swelled from five regulars to up to forty during the 40 Days periods, and she saw how distraught their presence could make patients. A priest led a group of protesters through the busy alleyway by the clinic, splashing what he claimed was holy water at passersby. Protesters would be up at the door, able to yell at and plead with patients until they finally made it inside. Some protesters would lie to patients and try to get them to park across the street at a Catholic ministry, rather than in the clinic parking lot. They would recite prayers on loop, yelling at the counterprotesters. One of the 40 Days for Life protesters even called one of Ulisano's Jewish compatriots an anti-Semitic slur. At one point, a protester brought a sign with the Nazi swastika symbol, waving it in front of patients' and the counterprotesters' faces.[19]

There was nothing Ulisano or any of them could do.

On the one hand, Ulisano understood why. The City of Chicago seemed to take the issue seriously. In October 2009, the city passed an ordinance similar to that of Los Angeles, creating an eight-foot "bubble" around patients within fifty feet of abortion clinics across the city. This bubble prohibited protesters from getting close to those approaching abortion clinics; the goal was to respect abortion opponents' right to protest while protecting patients from in-your-face harassment and possible harm.[20] City-area clinics hoped that this ordinance, like the FACE Act that preceded it, would cut down on aggressive antics. In theory, a clinic wouldn't need escorts if patients could enter the facility unimpeded.

But the increasing number of 40 Days for Life protesters, goaded by the legislative and judicial victories of the Bush years, proved no match for Chicago's law. The bubble zone wasn't going to enforce itself, Ulisano knew.

For two years, she and the rest of ICAT peacefully counterprotested at several Chicago clinics, standing off to the side, watching the bubble zone ordinance become another unenforced, empty promise. Every now and then, Ulisano would once again gently propose setting up an escort team with the clinics' staff. "Could we come on a more regular basis? I've trained escorts in the past. I *was* an escort in the past."

Eventually, Ulisano's warmth and dedication, along with the

escalation and endurance of 40 Days protesters, won some clinics over. In 2010, ICAT began escorting at several Chicago clinics. They had seen what 40 Days for Life was capable of, and now they would be able to protect patients on a more active, individualized level. Through ICAT, Ulisano created the first coordinated clinic escort team for the state in the new millennium.

It couldn't have come at a better time. By the end of the 2000s, 40 Days for Life had established itself as a serious, international antiabortion protest movement; leadership boasted protests at more than two hundred clinics in six countries.[21] Far from quiet, peaceful demonstrations, these protests—sometimes with hundreds of people—became a serious cause of turmoil and terror for clinic staff and patients alike. Mass protests were back, and once again, clinic escorts would form the front line of defense.

The Swarm Returns

The first time Autumn Reinhardt-Simpson drove by the Richmond (Virginia) Medical Center for Women in the spring of 2010, she was appalled by the scene out front. There was a mob of people holding bloody signs, and she could hear their screams radiate through her windows—"Don't murder your baby!" As far as she could see, there weren't any clinic escorts, giving the protesters unchecked access to each patient. It lit a fire under her, one that continued to rage weeks later.

The next time she happened to drive by the clinic, she felt compelled to stop. She parked her car and walked through the mob— who, mistaking her for a patient, begged her to turn around, told her that her baby would be ripped to shreds, that abortion was murder. She opened the front door of the clinic and asked if they had clinic escorts. When the clinic administrator replied that they didn't, she asked, "Can I be your one-member clinic escort team?"

Reinhardt-Simpson wasn't really sure what her offer even meant. She knew what clinic escorts were in the abstract, but she had never done it. She didn't know what it felt like, how to manage the scene.

When the clinic accepted, she dove in headfirst. She reached out to other clinic escort teams and asked for their training materials and guidance. Every chance she got, she talked to the people in her life about joining her. She read articles and watched videos.

Her first few times outside the clinic were a learning curve. At the beginning, she was the lone clinic escort, navigating roughly a dozen protesters at a time. She learned quickly: Stay close to the door. Greet patients warmly but not too giddily. Be a friendly face in a sea of angry ones. Remain calm. Don't engage with the protesters.

Then came 40 Days for Life.

The number of protesters would triple every six-week period that 40 Days came to her clinic. "It was shit for the patients," she said. It was hard enough weaving your way through ten people in your face; now you were facing more than thirty, all organized as a unit. This rapid increase in number was enough to intimidate some patients.

But it wasn't just the number of protesters that escalated; their behavior did too. What made matters worse was the way the different protest groups interacted with each other. The 40 Days for Life protesters were energized, and they in turn energized the other protesters. "The rhetoric amped up so hard. More people were very emboldened to yell things and yell more provocative things." Rhetoric like "Don't kill your baby!" was commonplace without the presence of the new protest group, but when 40 Days came, it took on a sharper, more religious tone. And it wasn't just what they said, but what they did. "They would follow [the patients] a lot more," she explained. "Luckily, we had our own parking lot [that was close to the clinic], but if people walked up from somewhere else, they'd follow them [to the clinic] for a lot longer."

Reinhardt-Simpson was nearly two years into her tenure as clinic escort and team organizer in 2012 when Virginia made national news. The state legislature, dominated by Republicans and led by a Republican governor, proposed a bill that required patients to undergo a transvaginal ultrasound in order to have an abortion, both medically unnecessary and incredibly invasive.[22] Suddenly, the issue of abortion was front and center in Virginia. Thousands of abortion rights supporters swarmed the state capitol in Richmond, demanding that lawmakers vote no. Late night talk show hosts lit into the legislation; Jon Stewart of *The Daily Show* called Virginia "the Punanny State" in a derisive segment.[23]

But for abortion patients in Virginia, it was anything but funny. While the capitol swelled with outraged abortion rights supporters, Richmond Medical Center for Women swelled with antiabortion protesters who were delighted by the newly restrictive environment.

Interestingly, Virginia Republicans proposed the transvaginal ultrasound bill in February 2012, right at the start of 40 Days for Life's Lent-season protest. Almost immediately, Reinhardt-Simpson noticed a serious uptick in protesters outside the clinic. The mood was different. It was more tense, more fraught. Patients seemed more tentative and afraid, she thought. "Besides the fact that you have all these restrictions . . . aside from that fear, more people were coming out to protest. You get more of *everybody* when [legislation like] this happens."[24]

One day that spring, in the middle of a deluge that included both 40 Days for Life and another fanatical religious protest group called Mount Gilead Full Gospel Ministries, Reinhardt-Simpson noticed a young Black man and Black woman walking up to the clinic, hand in hand. As she and another clinic escort tried to get to them, protesters quickly swooped in. The female protesters clustered around the woman and drew her away from her male companion, who had been surrounded by male protesters. Reinhardt-Simpson glanced back and forth at the two groups, unsure of what to do. The protesters had literally separated a patient from her companion and wouldn't allow them to reunite.

"The things they said were atrocious. To the man, [they would say, 'It's your seed.' [It was] couched in very religious, legacy kind of language. 'That's your seed! Don't kill your Black seed. Go in and take your woman out of there!' As if he had the authority to go in [and do that]. With the woman, they didn't let her speak. They literally just spoke at her continuously." By the time Reinhardt-Simpson had made her way to the woman, tears were streaming down her face. As she managed to get in between the protesters and the patient, some of the protesters began yelling in tongues.[25]

The combination of the tongues-speaking Pentecostal protesters and "sidewalk counseling" by 40 Days for Life protesters created a maelstrom from which abortion patients couldn't escape. While the media focused on Virginia's egregious legislation, it ignored the climate that already existed, and was growing more tense, at abortion clinics across the state. Reinhardt-Simpson began the decade as a clinic escort under the assumption that the last vestige of abortion opposition was the protesters at the clinics. What she and others hadn't anticipated was that movement translating into power at the state level. While Virginia's transvaginal ultrasound bill was roundly pilloried, the climate of fear and tension outside Richmond Medical Center for Women and other Virginia abortion clinics was left out of the national conversation. And while the national outcry forced Virginia's Republican governor Bob McDonnell to pivot, he refused to abandon the legislation entirely.

On March 7, 2012, as dozens of 40 Days for Life protesters laid siege to Richmond Medical Center for Women, just two and a half miles away, Governor McDonnell signed into law the bill that required providers to conduct a mandatory ultrasound on every patient before they could have an abortion, whether they wanted the ultrasound or not.[26] The message of this patronizing legislation, which spread rapidly to other states, was clear: people who need abortions can't be trusted to make their own decisions.

• • •

As the decade wore on, 40 Days for Life's numbers and targets continued to grow. By 2015, they had a presence at clinics in nearly every single state.[27] Clinics reported 21,957 cases of picketing and obstruction, a dramatic 288 percent increase from the year before.[28] This wasn't just in states that were dealing with restrictive legislation, like Virginia, but nationwide.

At both of the Chicago clinics that ICAT served, Ulisano felt the tension and aggression rise year after year. "It was very intense and the antis just kept coming . . . we [had to] guard the door. It was a very aggressive campaign." On any given day, the two Chicago clinics could expect roughly half a dozen protesters. But during 40 Days for Life, the numbers would swell to forty protesters at a time, and they were willing to test the boundaries of the FACE Act. "We're talking about people who were right up at the door, who refused to believe there was a bubble zone . . . Just up in our faces."[29]

During one 40 Days campaign, Ulisano was watching a large group descend on the FPA clinic when she noticed someone new. It was Ann Scheidler, the vice president of the now decades-old Pro-Life Action League, founded by her husband, the infamous antiabortion hero who helped pioneer blockades, Joseph Scheidler.[30] Ann Scheidler wasn't as hostile as her husband, but she refused to obey Chicago's bubble zone law. With dozens of people at the clinic day in and day out during 40 Days, protesters felt they had much more leeway to do what they wanted, especially with a lack of enforcement from local police.

For patients, that meant once again walking a gauntlet of people up in their faces, screaming at them and shoving gory literature at them. Ulisano and the other ICAT escorts began to see the limitations of traditional clinic escort tactics with the increasing volatility that accompanied the six-week siege.

The same was true of the nation's capital. The Washington Area Clinic Defense Task Force, WACDTF, one of the original clinic defense groups, had already embraced nonengagement at clinics in Washington, D.C. They saw a huge increase in protesters during 40 Days, as well as an escalation in aggression.

"At Lent, we get more and get more excitable people," explained Jemal Cole, a longtime WACDTF escort. "They are much more likely to be loud and try to engage with the patients. Some of them will bring a group of people and sing, some will bring children or toddlers. They'll hold them up and shout things about how that's a baby inside you, and they'll hold the baby as a prop."[31]

Cole and other members of WACDTF weren't just dealing with a yearly increase in 40 Days for Life protesters; they also had to contend with the growing "March for Life," an annual event in January in which hundreds of thousands of abortion opponents flock to the Capitol to protest *Roe v. Wade* and legal abortion. The march, which began in 1974, had more than 400,000 attendees in 2012. Five years later, that number would swell to 650,000.[32] The March for Life allowed hundreds of thousands of abortion opponents a unique opportunity to join an established protest effort at clinics around D.C. But that was a once-a-year event; clinics could plan for it, and clinic escorts could shore up their numbers. 40 Days for Life equaled eighty nonstop days of occupation.

As 40 Days for Life grew, so did other protest efforts. Perhaps fueled by the media attention, or simply reminded that protesting at clinics could still happen, other factional groups, like the Pentecostal church with which Reinhardt-Simpson tussled, organized their own protest efforts. Some decided to take it one step further.

Upping the Ante

In the early morning hours of November 9, 2016, what seemed improbable or even impossible had become real: Donald Trump had defeated Hillary Clinton in the race for president of the United States. The air was cool and crisp in Charlotte, North Carolina, that morning, a nearly perfect autumn day.[33] Near A Preferred Women's Health Center of Charlotte (APWHC), some of the leaves were turning the exact color the state had gone the night before: bright red.

Calla Hales, the clinic's executive director, was exhausted. She had barely slept that night. But that was nothing new for her. She hadn't been sleeping well for over a year. Since 2015, the clinic she runs, opened by her parents when she was a little girl, has experienced increasingly heavy protests from a group called Love Life. A cohort of dozens of area churches, Love Life took inspiration from many of the protest groups that had come before. As the Lent season approaches, clinics across the country annually prepare for six weeks of concentrated protests from 40 Days for Life. But not in Charlotte. Forty days feels like a pipe dream to the staff and escorts there. Instead, the Lent season marks the beginning of forty *weeks* of inundation and occupation from Love Life. For nine months every year, Love Life sets up shop outside APWHC.

Twice a year, Love Life stages large "parade days," in which a couple hundred protesters march up to the driveway of the clinic. They get a permit from the city to block off part of the road and essentially put on an antiabortion protest concert. These events, even though they are only twice a year, began to take a toll on Hales, the rest of the staff, clinic escorts, and most importantly, the patients.

Laura Reich, a sixty-year-old New York native, became a clinic escort that year. Her first day in December 2015 was a rude awakening. "As bad as I thought it was going to be, it was [so] much worse, because it was just all these protesters, screaming at these women and playing music," she said.[34]

APWHC was already home to some of the nation's most insidious antiabortion protesters, including Flip Benham, the leader of Operation Save America, a spin-off of Operation Rescue. Reich and the other clinic escorts at APWHC were accustomed to aggression and hostility outside the clinic's walls. Benham was the source of most of the escorts' ire—he was there day in, day out, and never seemed to stop yelling. As 2016 went on, Reich and others became accustomed to the tactics of Benham and the other regulars—how they would flirt with the limits of the FACE Act, how they'd try to intercept and deceive patients, the horrible slogans they'd chant. The clinic escorts developed their own tactics, learning how to spot patients and shield their faces from Benham's group with a large golf umbrella.

By the crisp morning of November 9, 2016, Reich and the others knew that things would probably get harder for abortion rights. Donald Trump would likely nominate Supreme Court justices who were hostile to *Roe v. Wade*, and abortion access would likely now be in serious jeopardy federally as well as state-wise. The one possible silver lining that existed: Republican presidencies often resulted in a decline in protest activity and violence at abortion clinics. Perhaps with a friendly administration in power once again, antiabortion protesters would take a bit of a break from protesting at APWHC.

What they found was a new reality. Instead of protests dwindling

under a Republican president, Donald Trump's election helped feed
what 40 Days for Life and Love Life had already started: a new level
of mass protests.

• • •

On December 3, 2016, Reich watched the sun rise over APWHC,
neon vest over her coat, icy hands wrapped around a warm cup of
coffee. She knew today was a "parade day," and she knew that Love
Life had claimed they would bring four thousand people to the clinic's front door. But the claim still seemed spurious at best. Love Life
had managed to bring hundreds of people to the clinic's driveway on
several occasions, but nothing near that many.

Still, as a precaution, twenty clinic escorts signed up for the
morning shift, up from the average of half a dozen.[35] The clinic
stationed defenders at the end of the driveway, holding big signs
that said THIS CLINIC IS OPEN and REJOICE IN CHOICE! They
even drew chalk arrows along Latrobe Drive pointing to the clinic
entrance.

That morning, Benham and a couple dozen followers were there
along with the usual Catholic "sidewalk counselors," one of whom
tried to direct patients into a nearby van that contained an ultrasound machine instead of the clinic.[36] The "regulars" were there,
calling clinic escorts "deathscorts" and holding their gruesome signs.
It was just like any other day.

Minutes later, a mass of teal emerged in the distance. As the blur
made its way up the street toward the clinic, Reich began to make
out bodies donning teal T-shirts over their winter gear. She tried to
estimate how many, but the group just seemed to go on and on. It
was clear this was no typical day at the clinic.

The chalk arrows along Latrobe Drive became invisible beneath the weight of more than two thousand antiabortion protesters, all wearing bright teal T-shirts. It was a mass protest unlike anything the clinic had ever seen.

While only half the number of anticipated protesters showed up, it was still a lively "coming out" party for the new group. Learning from groups before, they knew how to use the law against the clinic and patients by obtaining a parade permit from the city of Charlotte. They set up a stage near the clinic and were able to barricade much of the street. What looked like a "pro-life party" was really a de facto clinic blockade.

The clinic escorts were used to navigating fifty protesters, even a hundred. But they had never experienced anything like that first day.

"[There were] barricades, and thousands of people swarming," said Angela Anders, another APWHC clinic escort. "It took forty-five minutes to get up the street."[37]

As soon as a patient turned onto Latrobe Drive, they were stopped. Signs that read DON'T KILL YOUR BABY! and ABORTION IS MURDER! popped out of the sea of teal filling the street and sidewalks. Thousands of people were standing in the way of the patients' cars.

Traffic to the clinic was essentially blocked by the mass of bodies. Patients were frantically trying to find a way through as the minutes ticked by, afraid they would miss their appointments. The defenders at the end of the driveway tried to maneuver a way through the blockade to the patients' cars, attempting to direct them to the clinic's driveway. The clinic escorts, huddled together in the clinic's adjacent parking lot, would intercept the patients who were able to get through the logjam, shielding them as best they could from the parade pandemonium as they walked to the front door.

Once they made it inside, patients had to hear constant screams through the walls: "The devil hates you, and he hates your off-spring!"[38] and "Don't murder your baby!" echoing into the waiting room. There was no respite from the turmoil.

Abortion opponents were so pleased with the turnout on that first "parade" day in December 2016 that they decided to continue. While the parade could have been a FACE violation, no charges were brought, and Love Life would continue to adapt to ensure that they were technically abiding by the law while flouting its intention. Their next step upped the ante.

• • •

Nine constant months of targeted harassment each year have radically upended years of standard practice outside APWHC. The number of protesters didn't necessarily change the job of a clinic escort, but it made it more difficult for patients to even get to the driveway, let alone the door of the clinic. Volunteers tried to find ways to mitigate the terror and intensity that greeted patients during Love Life's presence. Even on less populous days, the mass of people can be jarring.

"For me as an escort, the difference between twenty and one hundred is pretty negligible," said Rachel Borsich, an APHWC clinic escort since 2017. "At that scale, my job is pretty much the same. I think it matters to patients. The more people on the sidewalk, the more intimidating it is. Especially when you get Love Life out there because they're bringing the numbers."[39]

"If you're coming when they're getting ready to do their walk, you see a mass of people crossing the street," explained Heather Mobley, another clinic escort. "You see a mass of people walking the loop and then ending up right in front of the clinic driveway."[40]

"Patients come in terrified," Reich said. "There's so many of [the protesters] and . . . a lot of times, when patients come in, they don't know who's who and what's what. They're terrified to get out of their car and we just have to talk them down and tell them to go inside."[41]

The clinic began to position volunteers more regularly at the end of the driveway, holding directional signs to help guide confused patients to the clinic entrance. "It's a game of chess trying to figure out how to best get patients in the building," Hales said. "If a car was stopped in the road, they'd say, 'The protesters are not with the clinic, keep going.'"[42] They also began engaging with the protesters, trying to distract them or draw their attention away from the patients who were driving up Latrobe Drive.

Love Life wasn't done finding new ways to antagonize the clinic, however. When the property next to APWHC went on the market, Love Life's leadership eagerly snatched it up.[43] This meant that the protesters were able to get much closer to the clinic's entrance than before, and Love Life could now center their parades directly next to the clinic. Thousands of people could be a stone's throw from the clinic entrance, gathered around the stage, enjoying an antiabortion protest disguised as a Christian rock concert.

Even more crucially, it allowed Love Life to ignore the recent noise ordinance passed by the Charlotte City Council, which prohibited amplified sound within one hundred and fifty feet of a medical facility, place of worship, or school, an all-encompassing means of curbing the absurd noise levels at APWHC without solely focusing on antiabortion protesters. But that law only applied to public property. Now that Love Life owned the building next door, they were no longer required to abide by it if they were on their own property.

Love Life is now the next-door neighbor of the abortion clinic it seeks to close. That proximity has helped reshape how Charlotte for Choice, the latest iteration of APWHC's clinic escort team, has approached protecting access to the clinic. Rather than simply employ nonengagement-based escorting, the team decided to try something different in an effort to beat back the forty weeks of misery: clinic defense.

• • •

When Hanna Roze decided to attend a training session for Charlotte clinic volunteers in 2017, she didn't know there was a difference between escorts and defenders. She listened as the organizer explained the divergent responsibilities of each position. Escorts were solely patient-focused and didn't engage with the protesters under any circumstance. Defenders were a relatively new role that they were testing out, tasked with directing traffic into the clinic and attempting to distract the most aggressive members of Benham's Operation Save America cohort and Love Life's massive throngs. Roze opted for clinic escort. She was glad she did.

She learned the ropes as an escort fairly quickly—always stay focused on the patient and never engage with the protesters. She greeted every patient with a warm and affirming, "Hi, I'm a volunteer with the clinic and I'm here to walk with you to the door, if you'd like." Once they said yes, she angled a large rainbow-colored golf umbrella to shield the patients. She used a calm, soothing tone when taking to the patients, aware that they were already hearing a significant amount of hostile noise and commotion coming from the building next door.

It wasn't just coming from the protesters; Roze became alarmed at the level of instigation that she saw from a couple of the defenders. She remembered one jumping in front of a car to physically block a sidewalk counselor from giving a flyer to the woman in the driver's seat. She was uncomfortable with the disorganization and feared that it would make it harder and more confusing for patients. "It was absolute chaos," she remembered.[44]

It became apparent very quickly that if APWHC was going to employ defenders, they were going to need to find a more strategic way of doing it. The physical tactics of clinic defense of the early 1990s—linking arms, literally blocking protesters with their own bodies—weren't working to put patients at ease or make entering the driveway to the clinic any less hectic. While massive protests were back, they didn't look like they had in the past.

Like Operation Rescue and other predecessors, Love Life staged massive events outside clinics. But unlike Operation Rescue, they didn't outright block the entrance. Instead, they used their carnival atmosphere to sow confusion among patients and make it harder, but not impossible, to get through. They used their numbers, rather than their physicality, as the deterrent. Nor did they park themselves in front of the clinic and refuse to move. Instead, they continually marched the loop around the clinic. They didn't stop moving, lest they be accused of a FACE Act violation. The simple presence of thousands of people, marching in a loop, was enough to intimidate patients. And because they owned the building next door, they could remain there, thousands of people camped out in front of a stage, without breaking the law. Love Life was able to flout the FACE Act without explicitly violating it.

Traditional clinic defense didn't work at APWHC. Matching the intensity of the protesters didn't actually work to keep the clinic open or help patients get inside. The challenge wasn't access, as it had been in the early nineties, but providing a more comfortable and straightforward experience for patients to get into the clinic. That wasn't going to happen by yelling at the protesters.

A New Kind of Defense

Benita Ulisano watched as the crowds at the FPA clinic in Chicago got bigger and more aggressive with every passing 40 Days period. "It was building, and building, and building," she said.[45] She and the rest of the ICAT members struggled to navigate the escalating levels of aggression with a strictly passive form of clinic escorting. The protesters were running roughshod over them—blatantly violating the bubble zone law by standing right up at the door of the clinic and getting up in the face of everyone who walked in the clinic's vicinity. Even the most confident, self-assured patients were wary and uncomfortable walking past the growing gauntlet—some literally ran toward the door.[46] Law enforcement refused to do much of anything—they seemed to loathe being called to the clinic and continually bucked having to enforce either the bubble zone law or the FACE Act. Finally, Ulisano had seen enough. She decided it was time to bring back repurposed elements from her clinic defense days in the early 1990s.

"Back then, we had to be very aggressive. Locking arms. Putting coats over people's heads and just being this locked arm of strength. [We had this] 'You're not going to get through us' kind of mentality . . . I said, 'We're going to have do a little bit of that.'"[47]

With the clinic's permission, ICAT began to integrate some old-fashioned clinic defense tactics, but with a twist. They once again formed a human wall, but without locked arms. Instead of planting themselves in front of the door, they became a mobile force.

"When we saw a couple coming and [the protesters] would try to do this gauntlet and follow them, there would be four ICAT people in between them and our patient, whether they liked it or not," Ulisano said. "This is what we have to do and that's what we did. Rather than block with our arms out, we would just waltz with someone but not touch them."[48]

The escorts wouldn't engage in lengthy conversations with the protesters, but they also wouldn't outright ignore them. When the protesters got particularly loud, Ulisano and others sometimes sang "Fa la la la la la la la la!" to distract patients from the cruel things that the protesters were saying. "Sometimes we use our Bluetooth [speakers] and that bothers them," she said. "When there's four of us doing that, it really drowns them out."[49]

ICAT's numbers continued to grow—Ulisano assigned more and more clinic escorts to the FPA clinic. Over time, they were so successful in shutting down the ability of protesters to target patients that eventually, 40 Days for Life stopped coming to that clinic. "We made our team so big that it was like, no, no, no, no, no—you are not going to accomplish anything here."

ICAT's integrated clinic escort and defense model worked to neutralize the unchecked ability of protesters to harass patients. Eventually, the protesters just left—until, of course, they showed up at another Chicago clinic. The game of whack-a-mole continued.

• • •

Calla Hales just wanted something that would work. Her clinic had become nationally renowned for the astronomical number of protesters they dealt with during parade days, 278 days of the forty weeks of Love Life occupation that made it impossible to function in any normal capacity. When the leaders of Charlotte for Choice approached her in 2017 with a different model for integrated clinic escorting and defense, she listened.

They proposed something unique: entirely separate duties occupied by entirely separate people in entirely separate areas. Up to six escorts, all clad in matching vests, remain on the property at all times and only interact with patients and clinic staff, providing an individualized support system for every patient and companion who walk from the parking lot to the front door of the clinic. Defenders, no more than five at a time, are off property. Rather than antagonizing protesters, defenders try to distract them with music or silly dances while directing patients to the clinic.

While they're very different jobs, at the core of both is one goal: to support the patient.

Hales decided to give it a try. The clinic had escorts for the six days a week that it was open, and they asked defenders to complement them on heavier days, typically Fridays, Saturdays, and particularly "parade days."

By 2018, Heather Mobley had two years under her belt as a clinic escort in Charlotte. She learned to use the simple tools at their disposal—large golf umbrellas, Bluetooth speakers playing happy music—to try to focus everyone she walked into the clinic on her, rather than on the screaming hordes mere yards away. "We try to calmly interact with patients, just try to make them feel like it's not as bad as it is so that they're calm going in."[50]

Mobley was frustrated at her inability to do anything to stop protesters from taking down the license plate numbers of every car that entered the driveway, a decades-old technique, originally from Joseph Scheidler's *Closed*, that abortion opponents have long used to intimidate abortion patients and doctors.[51] It irked her that patients were so confused and frightened by the thousands of teal-shirted Love Life protesters, that they had to navigate their way through a shame-filled party just to get to their appointment on time. More often than not, she found herself having to bite her tongue, to talk herself down, to keep herself from trying to intervene in a more direct way to keep the protesters at bay.

When Charlotte for Choice put forth a new kind of clinic defense, Mobley decided to give it a shot. She found it cathartic.

"We fully interact with protesters, even if it's drawing attention to us so they're not focusing on a patient or companion," she said. "[Patients and their companions] are in a stressful situation, and they don't need someone who doesn't know anything about their life screaming at them about how they're doing bad things. It's sometimes [about] getting the attention of that protester so they can't stay laser-focused on that [patient], even if it's yelling at [the protester]."[52]

Mobley and many members of Charlotte for Choice already knew the names of most of the regular protesters. She found that as a defender, one of the most innocuous ways to distract a protester as a patient was driving up was to simply call them by their name. They'd turn toward her while another defender waved a car past the protesters and into the driveway.

"They kill babies," yelled Ante Pavkovic of Flip Benham's Operation Save America. "They poison them, they dismember them. And then they say, as they wipe their bloody hands across their lying mouths, 'We've done no evil. We've done nothing wrong. We're helping people by murdering their offspring. We're helping people by killing little baby boys and girls.'"

"Hey Ante," a clinic defender shouted. "Do you like my shirt?"

"They hate the truth," responded another protester.[53]

Now, APWHC clinic defense is about distracting the protesters to mitigate their harm rather than lashing out at them. Clinic defenders speak back to them, but with a purpose: help the patient.

"The way we use defenders is more so patients have an understanding," Calla Hales said. "It has less to do with the protesters themselves and almost everything to do with the patients. That's the major difference between clinic defense twenty years ago and clinic defense now, is the fact that we're so much more patient-oriented rather than confrontation-oriented."[54]

Clinic defense doesn't stop the protesters from coming. It doesn't stop the cries of "Murderer!" and "Turn away from this evil place!"

from barreling through the walls into the waiting room. And it doesn't stop protesters from brazenly writing down the license plates of every car that drives up to the clinic or filming the people who walk toward the clinic door. It can't do that. It's not meant to do that.

It's yet another patchwork solution that has emerged to try to solve the often untenable situation outside APWHC. It isn't a perfect solution, but how can a handful of volunteers be expected to adequately neutralize thousands of protesters? In the end, clinic defense is meant to make it a tiny bit easier for clinic escorts to do their jobs—a job that shouldn't be necessary at all.

● ● ●

Decorative wreaths glittered on lampposts beneath the California sun. Bright white icicle lights flashed from across the street. All that stood between Cory Ellen and celebrating Christmas Day 2009 with her fourteen-month-old twins was just a few hours in a vest.

Ellen was fresh off six weeks of 40 Days for Life. Occasionally she was joined by one or two other volunteers, but most days, she was the only clinic escort on duty. Patients were initially confused by her—*Who are you?* their eyes asked. She would explain, "I'm with the clinic. I'm here to walk with you. I'm a clinic escort." They would soften and duck their heads while Ellen put her body between them and the 40 Days protesters.

Thankfully, the forty days had come and gone. She was still here. This pre-Christmas morning, like many that came before, she was on her own.

One minute, she was the only person outside the doors of Family Planning Associates Women's Health of Los Angeles. The next, she was surrounded by a semicircle of nearly seventy antiabortion protesters, many of whom were teenagers. At the center was a man named Jeff White, an extremist who founded Survivors of the Abortion Holocaust, the radical antiabortion group who was now face-to-face with Ellen.

Inside, the security guard watched attentively as the semicircle slowly closed in on Ellen. "They started caroling, creepily and aggressively and trying to get by me," she said. "Nobody touched me, but they were also really close, and I didn't know where it was headed, *and* I was alone . . . It was one of the most terrifying experiences of my life."[55]

For the next few years, Ellen worked tirelessly to make L.A. for Choice a full-fledged organization. What started essentially as a group of one blossomed to a rotating schedule of ten to fifteen escorts on any given day. Eventually, they added another clinic to their roster, and another. By 2013, Ellen was satisfied with the growth and stability of L.A. for Choice, and she decided to move back east.

"Clinic escorting means putting your body on the line," Ellen told me. "It means ensuring access and making sure that people can exercise a fundamental right."

Ellen doesn't volunteer as a clinic escort anymore. Instead, she's a registered nurse, working in labor, delivery, postpartum, and abortion. But back in Los Angeles, the bubble zone is still intact, and clinic escorts with L.A. for Choice, like Natalie Beach, are still ensuring that it is enforced.

"On paper, it seems like it should be easy and utopian," Beach said. She counts herself lucky, as the sizable crowds of Ellen's early days don't seem to be coming to the Family Planning Associates clinic where she volunteers, at least for now. "But even here in 'blue,' liberal Hollywood, you [still] have to get screamed at."[56]

Chapter Four

Last Clinic Standing

Isabel Valla (name changed for privacy) couldn't stop her knees from shaking. Maybe she just felt off for some other reason, she hoped. Maybe she was sick. Maybe this was somehow all a bad dream. Maybe, maybe, maybe. Valla had an intrauterine device (IUD), one of the most effective forms of contraception in existence. Somehow, her period was late. Then it was alarmingly late. Then she was peeing in a cup.

Valla was pregnant, an urgent care physician told her. Worse, she was potentially facing a nonviable and potentially life-threatening ectopic pregnancy, and she needed to go to the emergency room immediately. Whether it was viable or not, she knew she didn't want to continue the pregnancy. Before undergoing a series of tests, Valla told the doctor and nurses present that no matter what, she wanted an abortion. *These are medical professionals*, she thought. *If I want an abortion, they'll give me an abortion right here, today.*

She shifted in the ER exam chair, trying to get comfortable. Tears ran down her cheeks. How could this be happening? Grief and terror coursed through her body. One of the nurses walked in and Valla exhaled. Perhaps there would be a little solace in all of this, she hoped.

The nurse pulled up a chair, sat down, and faced Valla. "It makes me really upset to see you so sad when a lot of women would be happy," she said as Valla stifled a sob.

"It was jaw-dropping," recalled Valla. "I sat there, stunned for a moment and because of the shock of that, I didn't have a good comeback."

The nurse quietly left the room as Valla continued to cry. Her fiancé arrived in time for the tests to show that it was, in fact, a normal, viable pregnancy. The doctor handed her information on how to continue a healthy pregnancy and referrals for OB/GYNs. Valla wanted an abortion, something the hospital didn't do, and she wanted it today, something that Texas law, with a mandatory twenty-four-hour waiting period, forbade in 2015.[1]

"I looked at my fiancé and was like, 'What do we even do?' I had no frame of reference of 'Okay, I'm in hospital in [Texas] and I want an abortion.' Step one was just a blank. My fiancé said, 'All right, let's google abortion clinics.'"

Her closest options were Houston, Austin, or San Antonio, all over a hundred miles away. She chose the only one whose phone lines were still open that night: Houston Women's Clinic. The next available appointment wasn't until a week later, the clinic administrator told her. She would have to come in, fill out some paperwork, and then come back the next day, twenty-four hours later. Only then could she have an abortion. Valla made the appointment.

If Valla had faced the same situation just two years earlier, she would likely have had many more options for closer abortion clinics. Texas state senator Wendy Davis became a national star for her heroic thirteen-hour filibuster of Senate Bill 5, an omnibus antiabortion bill that, among other things, would force abortion clinics to meet the standards of ambulatory surgical centers and require abortion providers to have admitting privileges at local hospitals—both medically unnecessary and burdensome provisions designed to force clinics to close. Davis succeeded, but only in the interim. The bill was signed into law a few weeks later. By 2015, more than half of Texas abortion clinics had been forced to close their doors.

After booking a hotel room in Houston for herself and her fiancé, Valla had a frightening thought—*What if there are protesters at this clinic?*

There were.

As they pulled up to Houston Women's Clinic a week later, a dozen protesters gathered around their car. They held signs that said ABORTION IS MURDER with pictures of bloody fetal parts.

"We parked and got out of the car and all of a sudden, out of nowhere, that's when a clinic escort appeared," Valla remembered. "She was wearing one of the vests—I think it was rainbow—and had an umbrella because it was lightly trickling rain. I just remember that she was there, instantly, helping us out of the car and really quickly walking me toward the front door. I don't remember specific words. I know she was talking to me and that it was a pleasant tone of voice and reassuring. And I remember that she was physically standing on the side of me that was toward the protesters—she was between me and them. She was holding the umbrella over me and the feeling that I got was, this person is focused only on me right now."

Valla was luckier than many in Texas: She was able to take off work, she had a car, and she could afford a hotel room for two nights. At the clinic, she had a supportive partner and a clinic escort by her side. In the end, she was able to have an abortion and continue creating a life with her fiancé.

But the bill that Wendy Davis unfortunately failed to stop was now law, and it required every clinic that provided abortions to meet the standards of an ambulatory surgical center, a medically unnecessary provision that required clinics to either conduct significant remodeling, which could cost hundreds of thousands of dollars, or close their doors. This provision was one of several that became known as a "Targeted Regulation of Abortion Provider" (TRAP) law, which devastated abortion access across Texas and much of the Southeast and Midwest. Abortion opponents finally found something that could end legal abortion without overturning *Roe*: forcing clinics to close.

• • •

On June 27, 2016, Amy Hagstrom Miller sat in the hallowed halls of the nation's highest court, waiting to hear what was about to happen to her business. As the CEO of Whole Woman's Health, a reproductive health-care company with clinics in five states, including Texas, she was the lead plaintiff in a landmark lawsuit against the state of Texas for the 2013 TRAP law that forced Isabel Valla to drive more than one hundred miles for an abortion. The Supreme Court's decision today would determine what would happen to the three Texas abortion clinics she ran.

Just after 10:00 a.m., Hagstrom Miller emerged on the Court's front steps, wearing a crisp white blazer over a bright purple shirt. Purple had become the de rigueur color for abortion rights supporters during the oral arguments just a few months earlier.[2] Her right hand was raised in a triumphant fist.[3] They had won. The Texas law was unconstitutional. Abortion rights would live to fight another day.

In a post-decision press conference, Hagstrom Miller declared, "With this historic ruling, justice has been served and our clinics can stay open."[4]

Whole Woman's Health clinics did stay open, a significant victory. But after three years of fighting the TRAP law, dozens of Texas

clinics had already been forced to close, and closures weren't limited to just Texas. By the end of the decade, twenty-three states had
TRAP laws on the books,[5] and nearly a third of all abortion clinics
had been forced to close their doors.[6] If the Texas TRAP law had
been allowed to go into effect, the state could have been left with
fewer than ten clinics for 5.8 million people who might need abortion care, and those would have all been concentrated in the state's
big cities like Houston and Austin.[7]

A confluence of dwindling rural reproductive health care and
pernicious TRAP laws have created a new crisis for seven states:
only one abortion clinic left at all. By the end of the 2010s, a single
clinic remained in Kentucky, Mississippi, Missouri, North Dakota,
South Dakota, West Virginia, and Wyoming.[8] Some, like the Da-
kotas, had been hobbling along with one clinic well before 2010.
But most have seen abortion access ravaged by TRAP laws, and the
few clinics that remain are still fighting to keep their doors open
at all.

Having only one clinic to service an entire state doesn't just
make abortion harder to access; it makes it easier to target clinics,
and therefore easier to target patients. If there's only one clinic that
patients can go to, it's not too hard for protesters to figure out where
to go. Often, these protesters are heartened by the restrictions and
bans that conservative state legislatures try to impose. They see protesting as a means of ensuring that clinics close, one way or the
other.

The obstacles and challenges that plague other states—difficulty
affording the procedure, for example—are compounded by the fact
that in these states, there is only one place to go. The number of
patients at these clinics may be higher than at clinics in states with
greater access; because abortion is a time-sensitive service, the lone
clinic in a state being fully booked could mean having to wait longer

to have an abortion, increasing the price exponentially, or being forced to travel even farther to a clinic out of state. For abortion opponents, it's much easier and more effective to organize a large protest at one clinic rather than smaller protests at five. The last clinics standing are often inundated by both patients and protesters. And clinic escorts are stuck firmly in the middle.

Alone in a Crowd

For many North Dakotans, being alone isn't just a given; it's a perk. With slightly over 760,000 people, North Dakota's population ranks forty-seventh out of fifty-one, including Washington, D.C., averaging just eleven people per square mile. Being the only one around is normal. Being one of many is not.

Nearly 85 percent of North Dakotans live outside Fargo, the most populous city and home to the only abortion clinic in the state.[9] For pregnant people in need of care, that often means driving up to three hundred miles just to get to Fargo. For those coming from very isolated areas, where they are likely one of very few people, Fargo can be a culture shock on its own, even more so when patients have to walk through scores of protesters who know exactly where to target.

"This one couple walking into the clinic expressed concerns about the parking, and said she already felt overwhelmed being in Fargo," recalled Hilary Ray, who became a clinic escort in 2014. "This big town was already freaking her out."[10] Ray could feel this young woman's anxiety radiating off of her—she probably hadn't been around this many people in one place in a long time, let alone strangers who were yelling at her.

That sense of solitude and individualized I-can-do-it attitude is how Tammi Kromenaker is used to operating. A born and bred Midwesterner, Kromenaker spent nearly three decades of her life as one of very few people who work at the front lines of abortion care in the state. In November 1993, she got her first job out of college at Fargo Women's Health Center, then the only abortion clinic in the state. A week before she started, antiabortion protesters dumped cars without engines in front of the driveway of the clinic and two men occupied a welded metal box inside the car, in a bizarre attempt to blockade the clinic. Kromenaker pithily remembered how patients responded. "Guess what? Women have legs, and they just walked around the cars," she told me with a chuckle. "No one was denied."[11]

In 1998, Red River Women's Clinic (RRWC) opened its doors in Fargo, doubling the number of abortion clinics in the city and the state. Kromenaker was with RRWC from day one, eventually becoming the clinic's director. A mere three years later, she settled back into a familiar feeling: working at the only abortion clinic in North Dakota. Fargo Women's Health Center had closed its doors. RRWC was it for abortion patients in North Dakota.

Today, Kromenaker owns RRWC, running it with a sense of optimism and patience that belies the tenuous ground on which it stands in this conservative state. Years before TRAP laws emerged as an antiabortion legislative tactic, North Dakota was grappling with only one clinic to service patients statewide. Kromenaker has battled myriad restrictions to keep RRWC open, including a ban on abortions at six weeks (which was eventually blocked by a federal judge[12]), a TRAP law, and even a proposed "personhood" amendment, which would have banned all abortions and even some forms of contraception.[13] Her tenacious staff and supporters have weathered all of them, but there's one thing they can't overcome: the challenge of getting to the clinic in the first place.

• • •

For most of its existence, RRWC operated just fine without a need for clinic escorts. When the clinic first opened in 1998, it had a security guard, but once she was offered a full-time gig elsewhere, she left. *We don't really need anybody. We don't really have a problem*, Kromenaker thought. "It was the same old people from [Fargo Women's Health Organization] who would show up, we know all their names, it was the same."[14]

But after 40 Days for Life's first stint in Fargo in 2009, Kromenaker changed her mind.[15] She put out a call for escorts and, using training materials from WACDTF, led a packed room of volunteers through the training.

Kay Schwarzwalter was one of the volunteers. Born and raised two miles from the North Dakota border in the 1950s and '60s, abortion just wasn't a topic of conversation for her while she was growing up. Even after the Supreme Court legalized abortion nationwide in 1973, it remained a nonissue to her. But when a loved one told her that she was heading to "the big city" to get an abortion in 1985, she responded the only way she knew how: with unconditional support. "I don't know that my [loved one] told anybody else about this, but she told me and I was okay with it because I loved her, and I thought, she must have needed to do this."[16]

It would be nearly twenty-five years until she would really think about abortion again.

When she first began volunteering as a clinic escort, RRWC was once again in the midst of a 40 Days for Life occupation. Schwarzwalter threw a bright blue vest over her puffy parka, unaware of what to expect on a typically frigid November morning in Fargo.

She walked outside the clinic and was greeted with a cold chill and a jarring sight—a man stood before her, holding a sign that read KILLER HAD IT COMING. She turned her head and saw a priest, praying on his knees near the front of the clinic. "He threw holy water on us, whoever was in his way," she remembered. "He flung it all on us. I was just in shock, because I'd never seen [or experienced] anything like this."

That kind of behavior simply wasn't a common occurrence for Schwarzwalter or any other North Dakotan. In a state known for its "midwestern niceness," it was a rare sight to see a large group on a sidewalk, yelling at and accosting people, no matter who they were. It was a rare sight to see a large group on a sidewalk at all.

It soon became the norm on Wednesdays in downtown Fargo. It was the norm when Gary Lura started volunteering six years later.

When I spoke with him, Lura's midwestern niceness and sincerity practically jumped through the phone; he's "the sweetest, kindest man," according to Kromenaker.[17] He also defies every stereotype of a clinic escort or abortion rights supporter. Bald, five foot nine, and 225 pounds of pure muscle, Lura has, on one more than one occasion, been mistaken for a police officer by passersby.[18] His physicality and warmth lend themselves well to his favorite position, right by the door of the clinic, where he can see everything. More than anything, he's seen how the typical "midwestern niceness" can serve as a cover for the individualized harassment that accompanies the large crowds outside RRWC, especially toward men who accompany patients.

Positioned in his usual spot on an otherwise unremarkable Wednesday morning, Lura opened the front door to the clinic for a couple. The woman, young and quiet, walked in front of the man, who put his hand on the small of her back as if to say, *It's okay. You're okay.* Lura nodded at him as they went inside, then went back to monitoring the sidewalk.

Shortly after, the man walked out of the clinic alone. *Nothing odd about that,* Lura thought. Maybe he was going to grab a cup of coffee or have a cigarette. The man got a few feet away before a few female "sidewalk counselors" approached him, engaging him in conversation. Lura watched as the man's body language seemed to shift—he went from placid to perturbed. At some point, the woman he had arrived with came out of the clinic. *That* was unusual.

Finally, she was ready to walk back in. Lura opened the door for her, just like before, and smiled. As she walked past him, the man rushed in behind her. But this time, he wasn't playing the role of supportive partner. This time, he was desperate to stop her from having an abortion.

"He was having a bit of a heated discussion with the gal in the foyer there," Lura remembered. The man's voice rose and rose, and he began to yell at her to save their baby, to not commit murder. "I had the door open and just said, 'Hey sir, you need to come out,' trying to get him to come out [of the clinic]."

The man whipped around, pointed his finger in Lura's face, and continued to scream. "You're not going to tell me what to do!" he bellowed.

"I just stood there," Lura said. He used his physicality as a buffer, absorbing this man's screams, blocking the rest of the clinic from view. "And when he was done, I said, 'You gotta come out.'"

The man refused to move, refused to stop screaming. Eventually, another clinic escort had to call law enforcement to deal with the hostile companion.

It was exactly what the protesters wanted, Lura thought. These "sidewalk counselors" were nice and polite, warm and midwestern to this man. They used that "midwestern niceness," and the cultural reluctance of North Dakotans to be outright rude and dismissive of strangers, to convince this man that his partner was about to murder their child, when minutes before, he seemingly fully supported her.

"Some of these folks that don't really engage the patients that much, they might try and go and talk to the partner . . . There's a few women protesters that you might hear them talk to a partner: 'Go in and get her! Don't let her do that, be a man!'"

When I asked Lura whether the woman ended up having an abortion, he paused. "I don't actually know," he finally replied.[19] Whether she did or not, the clinic was able to continue functioning because Lura was there at the door. Other patients were able to have an abortion—at least that day, anyway.

• • •

While the protesters tried to disrupt the clinic in person, North Dakota lawmakers tried to do it through legislation. In 2013, the state passed a bill requiring abortion providers to have admitting privileges at a local hospital, but that wasn't all—that same year, Governor Jack Dalrymple and the North Dakota legislature shocked the nation when they approved a ban on abortions at six weeks, before many even know they're pregnant.[20]

Tammi Kromenaker didn't panic. Instead, she fought the ban in court, and she won.[21] As for the admitting privilege provision, she fought that too, and the law was blocked from taking effect. But she also organized and, eventually, reached a deal with a local health care group to provide admitting privileges to the provider at her clinic.[22]

Red River Women's Clinic would remain open for business, but it would also remain open to protesters. If the state couldn't outright ban abortion, protesters could make getting one as difficult and isolating as possible until the courts could catch up with the legislature.

They weren't the only ones.

Lighting the Fuse

Paula Schneider has lived her entire life in Kentucky. Born in 1948, she grew up on a small farm in a rural area just outside Louisville. The strict religious and moral code of her community dictated what girls like her could do and how they could do it, and it colored how she saw her own choices and the choices of other women. Her parents kicked her sister out of the house when she was just sixteen because she became pregnant, a reflection of the cultural attitude toward premarital sex and unplanned pregnancy. The messages of shame and stigma around sex were so ingrained as Schneider grew up that she didn't tell anyone about the abortion she had in her thirties while raising two kids as a single mother.[23]

When Schneider had her abortion in the late 1970s, Kentucky had seventeen abortion clinics.[24] By 1992, that number had been halved to nine.[25] Today, there's only one.

EMW Women's Surgical Center would be easy to miss if it weren't for one tell: the mass of protesters gathered at the entrance. The only abortion clinic in Kentucky is located down the street from Louisville's sleek conference center, right in the middle of at least half a dozen hotels. Tourists may be sitting on the balcony of their room at the Hilton and hear bellows of "Don't murder your baby!" ring out.

Since coming to full Republican power in 2010, the Kentucky state legislature, dominated by conservatives, effectively waged war on legal abortion across the Bluegrass State. In 2015, Kentucky elected a new governor, Matt Bevin, who made opposition to abortion rights central to his candidacy. Once elected, he delivered, and swiftly: Kentucky enacted a TRAP law that required abortion providers to have admitting privileges at local hospitals, an entirely unnecessary regulation that worked like a charm. By the time Paula Schneider turned seventy, there was only a single abortion clinic left in the state—EMW Women's Surgical Center.

Unsatisfied with having closed all but one clinic, Governor Bevin's administration repeatedly attempted to force EMW's closure through a series of sinister licensing regulations. At that point, the only thing keeping EMW open and operational was a series of federal court interventions—and a fiercely dedicated clinic escort team.

• • •

Meg Sasse Stern was just eighteen years old when she started clinic escorting at EMW in 1999. In 2007, she brought in a brand new recruit: her mother, Rita Sasse.[26] Since then, this mother-daughter team has seen 40 Days for Life emerge and set up shop. They saw the swell of protesters during the Obama years. Most horrifyingly, they have watched as abortion access has been completely decimated across the state. Their clinic has become an island, more difficult for patients to get to and easier for protesters to surround.

By February 2017, the outlook for EMW was bleak. Despite continuous court losses, Governor Bevin continued his relentless regulatory attacks against EMW in his quest to force its closure. The ACLU kept filing injunctions on behalf of the clinic. The doors stayed open, patients kept coming, and the Louisville Clinic Escorts still showed up, every single day, to ensure they could get inside safely.

A month earlier, Donald Trump had been inaugurated as the forty-fifth president of the United States. Here was a man credibly accused of sexual assault who, during his candidacy, claimed that women should experience "some form of punishment" for having abortions.[27] Not only did Trump's election increase mass protests at clinics, it spurred a new brand of radicals to raise the stakes.

Governor Bevin's repeated failure to force EMW's closure enraged abortion opponents. Somehow, with a far-right governor and far-right president, EMW still managed to keep providing abortions. The only way to make Kentucky abortion-free was to return to the tried-and-true tactics of old-school abortion opponents like Scheidler and Terry. The fuse had been lit.

On a quiet, chilly Saturday morning that February, Sasse Stern walked out the front door of the clinic and onto the sidewalk, orange vest shining brightly over her warm jacket. She looked around, doing her usual scan, until she noticed something different. There was the regular group of protesters that the team had come to know and begrudgingly anticipate, but on this day the sidewalk was littered with new faces. One of them belonged to Rusty Thomas, the new director of the radical antiabortion protest group Operation Save America (OSA), a spin-off of Operation Rescue.

Since Thomas began his tenure in 2014, OSA has galvanized abortion opponents into bringing back the days of clinic blockades and absolute disorder. While the organization is no longer under the leadership of founder Randall Terry, Rusty Thomas remains committed to employing the same kinds of tactics through OSA that made the organization's predecessor infamous: blazing well beyond the law in the effort to block clinic entrances and make accessing an abortion as painful as possible.

When Sasse Stern noticed Rusty Thomas outside EMW on that Friday morning, she knew something was off. She just didn't know what. It would be three more months until she and the rest of the team found out.

• • •

On Saturday, May 13, 2017, Erin Clark was up at 5:00 a.m. as usual. It wasn't hard for Clark to wake up that early. Clark (who identifies as nonbinary and uses the pronouns they/them) was used to it by now, and running a small farm meant waking up with the sun to get work done. They let the dogs out and handled some small farm chores before getting in the car by 6:00 a.m. An hour and fifteen minutes later, they parked and walked into EMW Women's Surgical Center for their regular Saturday morning shift.

When Clark got inside, the team threw on their orange vests and grabbed their last cups of coffee before heading out onto the sidewalk on West Market Street, ready to start. Clark stayed near the door with another escort, their preferred spot. Meg Sasse Stern took her standard post outside EMW on a nearby street corner. Rita Sasse was there too, positioned a block away from the clinic. Paula Schneider went to the other side, waiting for patients. Several other Louisville clinic escorts floated around, waiting for patients to accompany.

A woman got out of her car and craned her neck, looking for the front door. Sasse Stern was closest. She gently approached the woman and offered to walk with her to the clinic. The patient quietly nodded, and the two began what, for Sasse Stern, was a very normal walk. There was a regular protester or two who encircled them—"fruit-fly-style jabberers," as Sasse Stern called them—but that's why she was there: to be a protective extension for this young woman. "We were about halfway down the sidewalk by then, and I saw—you know when you see those pictures of bumblebee swarms? It looked like that around the door and property, but with humans, with all of their hands and phones up . . . I saw this entirely packed and swarming-with-people area near the door, and I pretty much immediately knew what was going on."[28]

Rusty Thomas was back, and he had at least one hundred other protesters with him. Three months earlier, Thomas had shown up at the clinic and made minimal noise. It became clear to Sasse Stern as soon as she saw the mass of bodies that morning that Thomas had actually been scouting the premises of EMW and making a plan for this organized protest effort.

Erin Clark and another volunteer stood on either side of the entrance. The clinic's front awning provided insulation from both the glaring sun and from OSA. Protesters almost never got that close to the door, avoiding a trespassing charge or, worse, a potential FACE violation. Thomas and a dozen OSA members then moved off to the side and huddled together. "They looked like cartoon characters trying to plan a heist with their whispers and sidelong gazes," Clark said.[29]

Almost as quickly as they had huddled, Thomas and ten other OSA members rushed up to the clinic, stood directly in front of the door, sat down, and refused to move.[30] The three-month-long fuse exploded into the first coordinated clinic blockade in thirteen years. OSA had come to Louisville to do what the Kentucky legislature couldn't—to close EMW and end access to legal abortion in the state.

Some protesters harassed patients and tried to disrupt access by blocking the sidewalk and flooding the surrounding streets. A few protesters wore orange vests, a flimsy attempt to disguise themselves as clinic escorts to confuse patients and companions who approached the clinic. Thomas and ten others occupied the front door. OSA members were everywhere. No one could get in—not even EMW employees.

The clinic was blockaded, and Clark and another clinic escort had become the only barrier between the protesters and the entrance. Not only could they not move, they knew if they did, the protesters would have unfettered access to the clinic.

"[We] were right under the awning," Clark recalled. "When they started coming up under there, we were like, 'We're not letting them into the door.' That's why we were under there; we were ready to move in front of the door and keep them from getting into the clinic. Both of us ended up not just against the door; we were pressed so tight, we had people sitting on our feet."[31]

With the door solidly blocked by a mass of obstinate bodies, anarchy was unleashed around the clinic entrance. Other members of the Louisville Clinic Escorts tried to figure out what to do; surely they couldn't walk patients through a dozen bodies barricaded against the door. The air filled with loud Christian music and bellows from the protesters, some of whom carried megaphones—"This is what pro-life is all about!" "Release this nation from this curse!" "This is murder!" "Each one of you are accountable to God!" "Matt Bevin wants to shut this place down. The governor has ordered this place closed!"

It was unlike anything Clark had ever experienced.

"It was scary. For ten of them to be completely, bodily on the property, obviously trying to get in the doors, and if they couldn't get into the doors, they were going to blockade," they recounted. "It was rough. It was really scary."[32]

To Sasse Stern, the sound was pervasive, a cloud of confusion and cruelty. The protesters' words zoomed by, ethereal daggers that weren't meant for her. She heard them but she didn't feel them. She was laser-focused on one thing: keeping them from hitting their target.

She knew there was no way in through the front door, but she also knew that she couldn't afford to panic. Any fear or negativity she displayed would only exacerbate the stress the woman she was escorting would feel. "At that point, it didn't make a lot of sense to turn around and go all the way back," she said. Instead, they moved off the sidewalk and into the street, shielding themselves from the mob with a line of parked cars. "I didn't want her to get noticed by more protesters." That meant potentially stepping into traffic. They attempted to loop around the back of the clinic through an alley to avoid detection.

Sasse Stern heard another escort's voice: "Meg, they're taking people in the back door!" She looked up and saw the clinic director standing in the alley, the rickety sliding gate that guarded the staff parking lot next to her ajar, as clinic escorts funneled patients through. The young woman with Sasse Stern mouthed "thank you" as she slid through the gate and approached the back door of the clinic. Sasse Stern reveled in the quiet moment of human dignity and connection for a few seconds, then walked around to the front of the clinic, back into the pandemonium.[33]

For the next few hours, Sasse Stern and her fellow team members spread out to find patients and loop them around to the alley in the back of the clinic, while the frantic scene at the front continued. Clark and their partner remained pinned to the front door for nearly half an hour. Somehow, in the middle of the chaos, a patient got stuck in the mass of protesters, and the escorts were unable to get to her. When the police finally arrived, they repeatedly asked each protester blocking the door to leave before forcibly removing them. Ultimately, eleven people, including Thomas, were arrested that day for trespassing.[34] Only then was the trapped patient able to get inside the clinic.

Every patient made it inside that day, shuttled through a literal back alley to avoid detection and danger, forced to walk past a rusted gate to get to their medical appointment on time. Patients were forced to go undercover, to stealthily sneak around as though they were committing a crime, simply to get inside a legal and reputable health-care facility.

Undeterred, OSA came back two months later, in July, determined to force lawmakers to "ban all abortions in the state of Kentucky," according to Thomas.[35] Rather than simply blockade the clinic, this time they held their annual conference in downtown Louisville, a spectacle of radical protesters who would inundate the clinic for an entire week. At times, the escorts felt it was like a morbid parade. "There were hundreds of protesters and lots of kids, walking up and down the streets," Paula Schneider recalled. "They had kids playing with chalk in the middle of the street."[36]

Armed with a temporary buffer zone from the Louisville City Council that barred protesters from being within eight feet of the clinic's entrance, the Louisville Clinic Escorts made some critical adjustments based on May's blockade. Instead of their regular orange vests, they opted for bright purple, hoping to avoid deceptive duplication by the protesters. The team also showed up even earlier every morning that week to beat the rush of OSA protesters. Once there, they made a wall of purple vests in front of the clinic, a tunnel of safety and security through which other clinic escorts could shuttle patients and their companions to the front door. It looked and felt like the early 1990s all over again, with one notable difference: this time, it was Kentucky's only clinic.

How Many Miles to Go?

The morning of May 21, 2019, another protest about abortion was happening in downtown Louisville. But it wasn't being held under the awning of EMW Women's Surgical Center—it was a mile away, outside the Romano L. Mazzoli Federal Building. And it was trying not to end legal abortion, but to save it.[37]

"Stop the bans!" the crowd of a hundred abortion rights supporters shouted. Some of the Louisville Clinic Escorts were there, wearing their bright orange vests. Free from the clinic's nonengagement policy, they joined the rest of the crowd in whistling and chanting to save the rights of the people they served.

It had been more than two months since Governor Bevin had signed into law one of the nation's most draconian pieces of anti-abortion legislation, a ban on abortions at six weeks, a point at which most people don't even know they're pregnant.[38] The ban, which was almost immediately blocked by a federal judge, never went into effect, and EMW continued to provide abortion care unimpeded.[39]

But by the time the crowd was shouting "Stop the bans" in Louisville, Kentucky's draconian ban had gone national. Following in its wake, six more states had banned abortion so early in a pregnancy that it essentially made abortion illegal.

The ink was still fresh on the unconstitutional Kentucky law when Governor Phil Bryant of Mississippi signed identical legislation.[40] Mississippi's only abortion clinic was once again directly in the crosshairs.

• • •

Michelle Colon was born and raised in Chicago, but Jackson, Mississippi, is home. Short in stature but big in energy and personality, she radiates confidence and cool, with a dash of showmanship. For the half decade she spent as a clinic escort at Jackson Women's Health Organization, Mississippi's only abortion clinic, she honed her unique gift of responding to abortion opponents with adept sharpness and shutting them down.

"Aren't you worried about the crime rate here, about your Black brothers and sisters in crime?" a protester asked Colon in a racist attempt to bait the biracial Black woman in the neon pink vest. "This is a crime!"

"Well, aren't *you* worried about the crime on my Black brothers and sisters?" she shot back. "Where were you at the last city council meeting?"[41]

That's what passed for a normal Tuesday at the clinic, what used to be one of the most unique abortion clinics in the country. Lovingly dubbed the "Pinkhouse" by supporters for its bright pink exterior, the clinic has been the last and only stop for abortion care in Mississippi since 2006.[42] Despite repeated attempts by state legislators to force its closure, it managed to remain until the Supreme Court struck down *Roe v. Wade* in the very case the clinic brought to the court, *Dobbs v. Jackson Women's Health Organization.*

The Pinkhouse wasn't like most abortion clinics, and it wasn't just the Pepto-Bismol pink that stood out. Most clinics have a rotating schedule of patients—you come at the time of your scheduled appointment. Not at the Pinkhouse. They booked patients in groups every three hours, beginning at eight in the morning.

But what was most fundamentally unique about the Pinkhouse was its now-extinct group of clinic escorts: the Pinkhouse Defenders. They yelled. They chanted. They held signs. They played music. They talked back to the protesters. They wore abortion rights gear like buttons and T-shirts. They engaged, and they did so proudly. They were unlike any other clinic escort team in America.

In their minds, they had to be. Mississippi is their home, but they also acknowledge that it is easy to characterize as deeply and intractably conservative. It's the most religious state in the nation: nearly two-thirds of Mississippians identify as "very religious," according to a recent Gallup poll.[43] The state hasn't had a Democratic governor since 2003. Fifty-nine percent of adults in the state say that abortion should be illegal in most or even all cases, the same percentage that identifies as "very religious."[44] Phil Bryant, Mississippi's governor from 2012 to 2020 and a staunch conservative, once called abortion "the greatest evil of our time" and a form of "Black genocide." Under his administration, Mississippi imposed scores of onerous abortion restrictions, including mandatory waiting periods and a TRAP law that required abortion providers to have admitting privileges at a local hospital.[45] The law was blocked by a federal judge, the only reason that the Pinkhouse was able to remain open until abortion became illegal in the state after *Dobbs*.[46]

But while abortion may have been electorally unpopular in the state, it wasn't uncommon. In 2017, about 2,500 abortions were performed in Mississippi,[47] and the state is one of the few whose abortion rates are actually rising—a 13 percent increase between 2014 and 2017, in the years *after* the state passed TRAP laws designed to close the Pinkhouse's doors.[48]

In every state, low-income women and women of color face barriers to accessing an abortion if they need one, but the challenges in Mississippi are compounded. The state ranks dead last in poverty rate,[49] and nearly one in three Black Mississippians lives below the poverty line.[50] Mississippi was recently ranked third from last in overall health care.[51] The maternal mortality rate in Mississippi is above the national average, but it's way worse for Black women, who are three times more likely to die in childbirth than white women in the state.[52] The patients at the Pinkhouse were mostly women of color, mostly low-income, and faced systemic barriers that make having a child exceptionally difficult. They made having a then-legal abortion nearly impossible.

• • •

It was a typical April day in Jackson in 2017, swampy and with little reprieve from the humidity. Derenda Hancock had already grown accustomed to the taunts of "Make America Great Again," in addition to the typical "Mommy, don't kill me, Mommy!" shouts outside the Pinkhouse.

Hancock noticed a car speeding up to the clinic entrance. The first group of patients had already entered the clinic an hour earlier, and the next group wasn't due for another two hours. The car, a jalopy in every sense of the word, had a duct-taped garbage bag as a backseat window and a small, misshapen spare tire on one front wheel.

Hancock slowly approached the car. If this was a protester, it was a sinister ploy to appear as if the people inside were patients. If this was a patient, they were incredibly late—perhaps too late to be seen. The cutoff for the 8:00 a.m. round of patients was 8:30, and it was now 8:47.

"Do you have an appointment?" Hancock asked.

"Yes ma'am," the driver replied. He gestured to the woman in the passenger seat. "It was at eight o'clock but we had a flat on the way here."

"Did you call the clinic to tell them you're going to be late?" Hancock asked.

"No ma'am," the woman in the passenger seat responded. "My phone's dead."

The young Black couple had driven more than two hours from the Mississippi Delta to get to the Pinkhouse that morning. Their two small children sat quietly in their car seats in the back. Hancock knew that if they weren't seen today, they likely weren't going to be seen at all. The clinic was booked solid for weeks.

Kim Gibson, a new member of the Pinkhouse Defenders, raced inside to alert the staff. Gibson had joined the team in the aftermath of Donald Trump's election, and while she was new to the role, she already knew the dire realities that many of the Pinkhouse patients faced. The clinic often tries to accommodate patients from the Delta because of the long distance and abject poverty that its residents face.

"Hurry! They'll take 'em!" Gibson cried from the front door.

Hancock leaned into the car and told the couple that the clinic would take them, but they had to hurry.

"I just need a minute," the woman responded.

Hancock could feel the seconds tick by. She heard the protesters begin to buzz anew.

"Let me live, Mommy!" "Don't kill your baby, ma'am!"

She glanced over and saw the couple frantically digging through the car's console and the glove box. Hancock panicked—what was she grabbing? If the woman had forgotten her ID, there was nothing the staff could do—she couldn't have an abortion.

Minutes went by. Gibson gave Hancock a look and pointed at her watch. They had to go and they had to go now.

"Excuse me, y'all, but we gotta get you inside or they're not going to take you," Hancock pleaded. The woman nodded and finally jumped out of the car. They began to walk toward the door, the sound of protesters filling the air around them. There was no music playing; it was the down period, between patient entrance and exit shifts. The woman was bombarded with cruel pleas and insults.

"We'll help you! You don't have to commit this grave sin!"

"Murderer! Murderer! Murderer!"

They were almost to the door when the woman stopped. "Ma'am?"

"Yes?" Hancock whipped around, trying to suppress her own exasperation.

"Will they take one forty-nine?"

"Excuse me?" Hancock asked.

The woman slowly opened her hand to reveal a wad of crumpled bills and a stack of coins on top.

"Will they take a hundred and forty-nine dollars? I'm a dollar short."

This woman and her partner had driven more than 150 miles, half of it on a spare tire, just to get here. She had scrounged everything she could find—a few dollars from neighbors, quarters from under the car seat—in the hope that it would be enough to afford a legal health-care service in her home state.

Hancock stopped. It was like the wind had been knocked right out of her gut. She took a breath.

"Sweetheart, I'm sure they will," she responded with her usual cucumber calm. "But let's just avoid that."

She pulled a dollar bill out of her pocket and placed it in the patient's hand.

The woman let out a small sigh. "Thank you so much, ma'am."

"Come on, sweetie, we gotta get you in," Hancock responded. She walked the woman inside, closed the door, and then turned to head back out onto the sidewalk.

"You don't have to murder your baby!"

"Your baby's blood is on your hands!"

"You have other options! You don't have to commit murder!"

Hancock closed the door behind the woman and whipped around. She glared at them, an all-white group of protesters, screaming at this young Black woman who had sacrificed everything to be here.

"You okay?" Gibson asked Hancock. She assumed yes. Hancock was always okay.

"No. I need a minute."

Hancock walked behind the clinic, away from the protesters and the people, and started to sob. She wept, alone, for the next twenty minutes. She thought of this woman, who was barely lucky enough to be seen today, who would have to come back for *another* visit just to have the procedure. And she knew that with the state of their car and their limited finances, the likelihood of that wasn't high.

Two and a half years later, Hancock was still emotional thinking about that couple when she shared that story with me. She told me what went through her head while she sobbed behind the clinic.

> I just sat there and thought . . . will they get back to the Delta on that donut? Because obviously, they don't have a tire. They can't even stop for a Coke. You know, all that digging in the car was digging up coins to make sure they had enough money for the first visit. And I won't ever forget that. That was the first time I was ever emotional at the clinic. That just tore me up. This young couple that are struggling so hard—they already have two babies. I don't remember at what point but he had said, when we were trying to get them in, he said, "Oh, ma'am, please. They really need to take us. I took off work to get here today." And all this was just running through my mind, how those—excuse my language—privileged motherfuckers on the sidewalk are screaming at this couple who did everything they could to scrape up enough money for the benefit of their family. They're having to go through all that plus this shit on the sidewalk? No. Just no.[53]

A week later, Hancock was back on the sidewalk, ushering in another 8:00 a.m. cohort of patients. The clinic was slammed that day—dozens of patients were filing in through the entrance. While helping another patient, she glanced over and saw that same young woman, back for her second appointment. She had made it. She was going to have an abortion. She was going to be okay, for today anyway.

• • •

On June 29, 2020, it had been exactly four years and two days since Amy Hagstrom Miller emerged victorious from the highest court in the land. She, like millions of others, sat looking at a screen, waiting yet again to hear from that same body on the exact same issue: an admitting privileges law.

Hagstrom Miller's victory was decisive and clear—the Texas TRAP law that forced Isabel Valla to drive more than one hundred miles to have an abortion was unconstitutional. But by the summer of 2020, the Supreme Court included Neil Gorsuch and Brett Kavanaugh, two new conservative judges appointed by Trump. This newly conservative court decided to take up a nearly identical law from Louisiana in *June Medical Services v. Russo*.[54] If the Court upheld it, the decisive 2016 ruling would be wiped away, and clinics across the South and Midwest would once again be in imminent danger.

When I talked to her a month before the ruling was released, Hagstrom Miller was defiantly upbeat: "I think hope is the biggest rebellion," she said. "We're in the business of second chances. People get to have these moments in our work that are beyond the political . . . how thankful people are, and how real those relationships are, that we really help people get the care that they need and step back into the life they dreamed of. It's pretty rewarding. That's where the hope comes from."[55]

In the end, her hopefulness was rewarded, albeit tepidly. The Supreme Court narrowly ruled the Louisiana law unconstitutional, allowing clinics to remain open in the state. But it did leave the door open for other restrictions. As clinic escorts and staff in one-clinic states have seen, hostile legislators keep finding more and more creative ways to close their doors. For the moment, disaster had been averted. That was something, at least.

Hagstrom Miller's neighbor and fellow abortion provider Tammi Kromenaker has the same sense of optimism, one that has been thoroughly tested over the previous decade. "I just really love my job," she answers when asked why she keeps going.[56] She's fought TRAP laws, severe abortion bans, and thousands of protesters with a smile on her face masking the grit in her teeth. For nearly twenty-five years, Red River Women's Clinic was North Dakota's sole abortion clinic. Now that *Roe v. Wade* has been struck down, and facing North Dakota's trigger law that will make abortion illegal, Kromenaker is once again relying on that grit to move her clinic a ten-minute drive across the river to Moorhead, Minnesota, where abortion is more likely to remain legal

Gary Lura plans to continue volunteering. "As long as I'm able to," he said. "I believe in the ability to choose."

Chapter Five

From Bombs to Bans

MAY 19, 2019, MARKED ONE YEAR SINCE TAMARA SOROKO had moved back to her hometown of Birmingham, Alabama, but she wasn't in the mood to celebrate. There was no toast or party. Instead, she was doing exactly what she had been doing thirty years earlier: fighting to keep abortion accessible in her home state.

Initially, Soroko didn't want to move back to Birmingham. Growing up in "Bombingham," as it came to be known for the frequency of white supremacist bombings during the civil rights movement, Soroko was just a girl when four Black girls were killed after a bomb went off at the 16th Street Baptist Church in 1963. She was still a girl when she was raped by a family member. As a young adult, she had an abortion, and later she became a clinic escort during the heyday of Operation Rescue. Birmingham was a site of trauma and painful memories.

She and her husband were perfectly content to remain living in the Pacific Northwest, amid the frequent rain and more relaxed social mores. When she thought of Birmingham, she'd once again see the hand reach toward her neck. She'd feel the weight of dozens of bodies pressing against her. Screams of "Murderer! Rot in hell!" would ring in her ears.

But her father was aging, and he needed her. In May 2018, after eight years away, Soroko was once again an Alabama resident.

A year later, she was marching through downtown Birmingham alongside scores of other abortion rights supporters, decrying the state's newest law: a total ban on abortion, punishable by up to ninety-nine years in prison.[1] It was the most draconian and restrictive abortion ban in the country, and if it were allowed to go into effect, it would completely end legal abortion in the state.

As the group made their way down the streets of her hometown, she felt the familiar wisps of déjà vu. The sight of a hundred people lying across the sidewalk. The woolen scratch of a scarf against her hand as she threw it over a woman's head. The chants of "My body, my choice!" fading into "Don't kill your baby!"

It had been more than thirty years since Soroko flipped on the local news to see over a hundred Operation Rescue protesters blockading Birmingham's New Woman, All Women Health Care clinic, part of a coordinated blockade effort across the country. Fresh out of the shower, she hopped in her car, drove to the clinic, threw on a vest, and joined the burgeoning clinic defense movement against Operation Rescue.

Soroko knew firsthand how hard they had to fight to keep the clinic open during Operation Rescue's reign of terror. She used to walk through "a literal tangle of bodies," tip-toeing through the protesters strewn across the pavement, trying not to step on them. When a patient expressed fear, she would drape her wool scarf over their heads to shield them from the protesters. Sometimes she had to get physical.

"As I got to the tangle of bodies . . . I started bulldozing my way through. I put my fists to my face and elbows out and started pushing through. I actually saw hands reaching through bodies and coming to my neck. They wrapped around my neck and started shaking me.

I don't know who those hands were attached to, but I screamed, 'Some Christian is choking me!' And they stopped."[2]

In its immediate aftermath, the FACE Act of 1994 helped mitigate some of the worst behavior outside New Woman, All Women Health Care, ending blockades and seemingly removing the need for clinic escorts and defenders. But that sense of safety was shattered on January 29, 1998, when Eric Rudolph, a domestic terrorist who previously bombed the opening ceremonies of the 1996 Olympics in Atlanta, successfully detonated a bomb inside the Birmingham abortion clinic. Robert D. Sanderson, the clinic's security guard who had tried to fix a misplaced plant that contained the incendiary device, was killed.[3] Emily Lyons, the nurse who opened the clinic, was severely injured and left permanently blind. She later described what the bombing did to her: "I lost my left eye, it damaged my right eye, broke the right side of my face, first-, second-, and third-degree burns on the front of my body, broke my leg . . . tore the muscle and skin right off the front of my leg, hole in my abdomen—my intestines were hanging out."[4]

This, the first fatal bombing of an abortion clinic in U.S. history, shook more than Birmingham. For Tamara Soroko, it felt like Rudolph had blown up the legacy she had tried to leave at New Woman, All Women just a few years earlier. By then, Soroko was already living out west. The clinic would reopen, and it would continue serving patients for another fourteen years until it was forced to close in 2012 after a losing battle to renew its license with state regulators.[5] Birmingham has been without an abortion clinic ever since.

But when Soroko came back to Birmingham in 2018, she had no idea how quickly she would be thrown back into the fight. By 2019, facing illegal and criminalized abortion for the first time in forty-six years, Soroko once again felt like she was being choked. But this time, it wasn't by a protester; it was by the state.

• • •

The passage of Alabama's total abortion ban was the eventual apex of a year filled with abortion bans. By the time Republican governor Kay Ivey signed that ban into law in 2019, three states—Georgia, Mississippi, and Kentucky—had already banned abortion at six weeks, which served as de facto total abortion bans, since it's before most people are even aware that they're pregnant. By the end of 2019, five more states banned abortion earlier than *Roe v. Wade* allows.[6] The wave of abortion bans seemed unstoppable, with the federal courts left to serve as last finger in the dike—none of them were allowed to go into effect. None of them were meant to go into effect. They were passed with the explicit knowledge that they were unconstitutional. The hope was that with Brett Kavanaugh's 2018 appointment to the Supreme Court, these state-level bans could finally lead to the antiabortion movement's ultimate goal: the overturning of *Roe v. Wade* and an end to nationwide legal abortion.

While these laws worked their way up to the Supreme Court, abortion remained legal in each of these states, and their clinics stayed open. The bans themselves didn't end abortion, but they could curtail it in a particularly sinister way—scaring pregnant people into thinking that it was now illegal. If patients still showed up at clinics, they'd be met with an emboldened antiabortion protest movement that, believing they were on the verge of the end of *Roe*, recommitted itself to being even bigger and more intimidating than before.

They would also be greeted by a friendly face with a neon vest who knew that it was more important than ever to support someone who needed an abortion. Clinic escorts couldn't stop abortion bans, but they could support this right in a more individualized way. They knew they had to, because just like in the early 1980s, they knew that no one else would.

An Old Fight Made New

The Ohio Statehouse atrium's front glass doors were foggy from dozens of warm breaths, smeared with fingerprints of anger and aggression. The doors were locked the morning of April 13, 2020—shuttered in response to a devastating pandemic—and a hundred vitriolic Trump supporters were demanding that they reopen.

Republican Ohio governor Mike DeWine had become persona non grata for many conservatives after he imposed a strict "stay-at-home" order and ordered the closure of all nonessential businesses to stem the tide of the coronavirus pandemic.[7] The protesters gathered in front of the statehouse, almost none of them wearing masks to prevent the spread of the virus, angrily demanding that he reverse course.

Michelle Davis decided to drive by the protest to see what was happening. She took a camera with her and sat in her car, photographing the event. She scanned the crowd, pointing and shooting, until she came across a middle-aged man with a long gray beard, wearing a saggy, white-collared shirt and black baseball cap, surrounded by a group of far-right extremists who called themselves the "Boogaloo Boys."[8] She knew his face instantly. It was John Brockhoeft, and he was no stranger to the far-right.

In the early morning hours of December 30, 1985, while many Cincinnatians were still sleeping off another night of a warm holiday season filled with loved ones, Brockhoeft was alone, covertly ping-ponging between two abortion clinics in downtown Cincinnati.[9] Both would be in flames before the night was over. One of the clinics, a Planned Parenthood, burned to the ground.

Then mayor of Cincinnati Charles Luken called it "terrorism in our community."[10] It would be another two years until the Planned Parenthood would reopen. It wasn't until 1991 that Brockhoeft was finally sentenced to seven years in prison for the firebombing, and only after he was sentenced to twenty-six months for another crime—planning to bomb the Ladies Center in Pensacola, the future site of three antiabortion murders.[11]

Brockhoeft was unapologetic in the aftermath of his own sentencing: "I put myself in the baby's place, reminding myself that I had to love that baby as myself . . . If I, like the baby, was going to suffer so much and then die tomorrow morning, and I knew I was being killed unjustly, I would not be too afraid to go to the death chamber with gasoline and destroy it tonight."[12]

Now, amid the most devastating pandemic in a century, this man was leading protesters, many of whom were armed, to the front steps of Ohio's capitol, decrying the stay-at-home order as a violation of privacy and liberty. But just one year earlier, in April 2019, Governor DeWine became a bona fide hero to abortion opponents when he followed in the neighboring state of Kentucky's footsteps, signing into law a ban on abortions at six weeks.[13] That ban, the culmination of years of work to curtail abortion access in the state, was blocked by a federal judge. But it still signified a victory for abortion opponents—the more opportunities they could give the Supreme Court to overturn *Roe v. Wade*, the better. It also reenergized those who were still protesting at abortion clinics, believing that the law might soon be on their side.

• • •

On the morning of Tuesday, May 7, 2019, Helmi Henkin was where she usually was: outside West Alabama's Women Center in Tuscaloosa. One of the three remaining abortion clinics in the state and the only clinic in western Alabama, the clinic had survived a 1997 firebombing, a car careening through its doors in 2006, and, more recently, TRAP laws and licensing threats by hostile state lawmakers.[14]

Now those very same lawmakers were debating a new bill that, if passed, would outlaw abortion entirely and serve as the strictest abortion ban in the country.

The clinic is just across the highway from the University of Alabama, and that proximity has helped keep the clinic alive through decades of protests and violence. Staff and students at the university have a front-row seat to the toll that daily protests take at the clinic. They have formed the backbone of the West Alabama Clinic Defenders, the clinic's escort group, and as the state has moved to outright ban abortion, they have seen the cost of that escalation at the very doors they are trying to protect.

Henkin, whose wide smile and long, flowing blonde hair can sometimes mask her fearlessness and commitment, started volunteering as a clinic escort in October 2016. She was instantly hooked, drawn to the marriage of one-on-one compassion and tenacious bravery. Her calling was to help people, she reasoned, and there was no more concrete way to do that than to walk people in when they needed support. While many of her classmates were sleeping off a hangover from the night before or getting an early start for a Crimson Tide football game, Henkin woke up every Saturday morning before sunrise, grabbed a cup of coffee, and drove in the opposite direction of the stadium to the West Alabama Women's Center.[15]

It has never been easy to be a clinic escort in Alabama, but Henkin and the West Alabama Clinic Defenders fell into a relative groove. They knew who the recurring protesters were and how to mitigate their tactics. Violence didn't feel like a pressing threat.

But in the fall of 2018, Henkin felt a shift. That November, Alabama voters approved an amendment to the state constitution to equate fetuses with people, eradicating the right to an abortion in the state. That law is currently superseded by federal law, but if the Supreme Court ever does overturn *Roe v. Wade*, abortion will become instantly illegal in Alabama.

Not content to rest on their antiabortion laurels, Alabama conservative lawmakers upped the stakes in the spring of 2019 when they proposed the total abortion ban against which Tamara Soroko would soon march in protest. It was then that the climate outside West Alabama's Women Center took a decisive turn.

That warm May morning, as Alabama state senators were beginning their debate on this unprecedented abortion ban, Henkin was already sweating through her rainbow clinic escort vest under the scorching Alabama sun when she noticed a Toyota SUV, spray-painted black, pulling into the parking lot.[16] Along with her sixty-five-year-old fellow clinic escort Jamie Johnson, Henkin approached the car. Henkin quickly recognized the man behind the wheel. He was neither a patient nor a companion—he had been there before, in the exact same car, doing the exact same thing. He first showed up in February 2019, circling the parking lot while verbally taunting clinic escorts.

"He came barreling into the lot in his matte-black SUV, threatening to hit us," Henkin recalled. "He showed up sporadically, on Saturdays mostly, and would do slow donuts in the parking lot around patients' cars, letting us know he was watching."[17]

He was back this morning, idling in the parking lot while chatting with a protester, essentially blocking the driveway, which was a FACE violation. Henkin and Johnson walked over to film him, documenting the violation, when he began to back his car in their direction. He had threatened them before, but it had never been physical. Surely he would stop before he reached them.

But he didn't stop. He backed his car directly into Johnson, hitting her in the side and running over her foot.

"You just hit me!" she yelled, in complete shock.[18]

"Move, you fat-ass bitch, or I'll hit you again!"

Henkin helped an injured Johnson move out of the way before he sped off.[19] Johnson had minor injuries but was otherwise okay. Henkin's usual bright smile was erased by tears of anger and outrage.

Henkin called the police, and the Tuscaloosa Police Department recorded the incident as a "hit-and-run involving a vehicle driven by a white male."[20] But in Henkin's view, it was yet another example of law enforcement failing to take seriously the aggression—and in this case, the outright violence—outside abortion clinics. According to Henkin, the magistrate who watched the video of the incident chastised the clinic escorts for walking toward the car in the first place before throwing the case out.[21]

Both Johnson and Henkin were back in their vests the next day, walking patients in. "These men are not going to silence this voice now that I've found it," Johnson defiantly declared.[22]

Henkin was there a week later, on May 16, when Governor Ivey made performing an abortion in the state of Alabama a felony punishable by up to ninety-nine years in prison. Abortion wasn't illegal yet—the law wouldn't take effect for six months[23]—and patients, after being reassured by clinic staff that their appointments were still on, still showed up. They still had to make their way past a group of protesters, many of whom screamed at them that they were evil sinners but refused to condemn the man who had run over a sixty-five-year-old woman with his car. Henkin knew that he could come back. She knew that it was possible, even probable, that something similar would happen again. The protesters were jubilant at the passage of the total abortion ban, and in the meantime, until the ban was either allowed to take effect or worked its way up to the Supreme Court, they could deter abortion in a more direct way. The West Alabama Clinic Defenders couldn't sue to block the ban, but they could shield a patient from an angry, hateful man screaming that she was a "je-zebel." It was clear the clinic escorts couldn't stop showing up. The need was too great, and the response from law enforcement wasn't strong enough to deter outright attacks on clinic escorts' lives. This time, the attack was by car. Next time, it could be a return to the old: it could be a fire, or a bomb, or a gun.

"People often say that clinic escorts are heroes and thank us for being out there and they call us brave," Henkin said. "I appreciate their comments, but it doesn't always register to me how courageous what we're doing actually is because I did it almost five days a week for three years. Stuff like that is a reminder that we're really putting our lives on the line."[24]

The Deception Inception

For the past few years, the sound of a phone ringing has been the easiest way to get Michelle Davis's attention. To the thirty-nine-year-old, that ring usually means someone needs help.

"Hello, you've reached Women Have Options. This is Michelle, how may I help you?"

Since 2018, Davis has run the patient hotline for Women Have Options, a nonprofit organization that provides financial assistance to people in Ohio who need an abortion but can't afford one. While Ohio is technically a "swing state," it hasn't had a Democratic governor since 2011, and the years since then have been filled with abortion restrictions and bans. Ohio clinics were closing left and right, devastating access. By 2017, 93 percent of Ohio counties lacked an abortion provider. The TRAP laws championed by Governor John Kasich worked. In December 2016, Kasich vetoed a six-week abortion ban in favor of a less draconian, yet still unconstitutional ban at twenty weeks. On top of that, the state does not provide Medicaid funding for abortion care, and it bars private insurance purchase through the Affordable Care Act exchange from covering abortion, as well.[25] The result is that for many, a common procedure is entirely unaffordable.

That's where Women Have Options comes in—they help fill the financial gap that Ohio's restrictions create. Davis received calls from pregnant people who were unsure of where to go for an abortion or how they would pay for one. She's a fountain of information and support, because she doesn't just run the Women Have Options hot-line; she's also a clinic escort, and she has been where these patients have been.

"I had my oldest child, who is now a sophomore in college, when I was in high school," she recalled. "I became pregnant again when I was nineteen and I knew I was not ready to have another kid. I knew I was going to have an abortion. There was no doubt in my mind. I just had to come up with the money."[26]

As the hotline operator, Davis could help someone pay for an abortion on Monday and then greet them on Saturday at Your Choice Healthcare in Columbus, one of the handful of abortion clinics left in Ohio. She felt increasingly confident that she could handle nearly any question that a caller would ask.

But in April 2019, a caller posed a new question, one that stopped her in her tracks.

"I'm pregnant but I think I'm over six weeks. Is it still possible for me to get an abortion in Ohio? Are the clinics all closed?"[27]

It wasn't true. But Davis knew why the caller thought it was.

On April 11, 2019, Governor Mike DeWine signed into law a ban on abortions at six weeks, joining other conservative states like Kentucky and Georgia. He championed the bill, entitled the Human Rights Protection Act, as a measure that would "protect those who cannot protect themselves" before openly admitting that it was intentionally unconstitutional to provoke the Supreme Court to overturn *Roe v. Wade*.[28]

To Davis, those words weren't just hollow; they were hypocritical. Though the ban was never able to take effect—it was soon blocked by a federal judge—many callers didn't understand that. They simply saw "Ohio bans abortions" on the news or social media and thought that meant that abortion was now illegal in their state. The six-week ban wasn't protecting anyone, Davis thought. It was scaring and even deterring those who needed care from seeking it.

That wasn't an accident. That was the point.

• • •

By April 2020, it had been weeks since Kristin Hady had been able to clinic escort at Capital Care in Toledo, Ohio. It wasn't because she was too busy—she had more flexibility in her schedule than ever. Because she helped care for her husband's parents, one of whom was in at-home hospice care, she couldn't risk their lives with potential exposure to COVID-19. Her vest remained tucked away in a locker, gathering dust.

The pandemic upended every aspect of everyone's lives. Suddenly, you couldn't be within six feet of another person without risking their lives and your own. Schools were shuttered. Restaurants were closed. Libraries, coffee shops, museums—every public door was suddenly closed across the United States, and most of the world. Cities like New York, meccas of culture and energy, were dormant, except for the constant blare of sirens.

Without any coordinated, competent federal response from the Trump administration, states were left to their own devices. Those with Democratic governors, in particular, issued strict "stay-at-home" orders, requiring everyone to shelter in place and avoid going to public places except for critical services like groceries or medical care. Most states with Republican governors followed the topsy-turvy, anti-science lead that the president had established. But a few, like Ohio, bucked that trend and took the pandemic, which would end up costing hundreds of thousands of American lives, seriously. .

On March 15, 2020, Governor DeWine issued a "stay-at-home" order for Ohio, forcing all nonessential businesses to close.[29] The order didn't apply to health-care facilities, so abortion clinics remained open. With bans on gatherings of more than ten people, it was exceptionally difficult for some clinics to even keep their escort programs going and still abide by the order. Technically, as agents of the clinic, clinic escorts could still be there, but the risk of exposure for themselves, their families, and the patients they served seemed too great for most teams to continue, at least in the early weeks of the pandemic.

With the coronavirus as its excuse, the DeWine administration tried to chip away at abortion yet again. On March 17, the Ohio deputy attorney general demanded that abortion clinics stop performing "nonessential" abortions, citing Ohio health director Amy Acton's previous order halting all "elective" procedures.[30] It was a sinister ploy, using the pandemic as cover to try to stop legal abortions in the state.

For a state that just a year earlier had tried to ban abortions at six weeks, it seemed clear that the goal wasn't to "preserve PPE (personal protective equipment)" for frontline health-care workers but to delay abortions, potentially past the point of legality.[31] It was, in essence, a backdoor abortion ban.

Ohio clinics like Kristin Hady's own Capital Care fought back, asserting that abortion wasn't like other elective procedures in that it was both time-sensitive and essential care.[32] They filed suit to keep their doors open. A federal judge overruled Ohio's order, and abortions were able to continue.[33] But the media coverage around that order, coupled with the six-week ban that never actually went into effect, created a climate of bewilderment for many who needed abortions in the state. "I think people definitely thought that abortion was not going to be accessible," Davis said. "That was a constant issue, and it was very hard to explain because it's so convoluted."[34]

When operating the hotline, Davis continued to reassure callers that yes, abortion was still legal in Ohio, and yes, clinics were still open and operating, even in the middle of COVID-19. It just looked different for patients now; to cut down on traffic and exposure, they couldn't bring a support person in with them, and they had to wear a mask at all times.

Outside the clinics, however, it was easy for patients to assume— at least initially—that nothing had changed at all. Protesters were still at Capital Care in Toledo and at Your Choice Healthcare in Columbus. Almost none of them wore masks.

Just like severe early abortion bans, Ohio's idea quickly spread among conservative states. Within a month, ten more states had joined Ohio's attempt to ban abortions as elective procedures during the COVID-19 crisis, including states that had already passed draconian abortion bans, like Mississippi and Louisiana.[35]

It happened in Alabama, too. Bianca Cameron-Schwiesow wasn't surprised. After years volunteering as a clinic escort in Alabama, she knew that anti-choice legislators in the state would find a way to use this pandemic to their advantage. Like Ohio's COVID-19 ban and its very own abortion ban, Alabama's COVID-19 ban wasn't allowed to go into effect, and legal abortions continued.

It was a cloudy and humid morning on May 18, 2020, and clinic escorts gathered at Reproductive Health Services, an abortion clinic in Montgomery. A year earlier, they had seen how an abortion ban could rile up aggression and even violence from protesters. Now, yet another attempt to ban abortion in their state had fallen flat, and patients still needed to get inside. Despite the tragic stakes that COVID-19's escalating death toll revealed, protesters were still outside. Was it a greater risk to escort or a greater risk not to?

They decided to try. They suited up, pulling rainbow vests over their bodies and securing cloth masks over their noses and mouths, and walked out into the muggy May morning.

Cameron-Schwiesow stood by the clinic's front door, waiting and watching. She saw the group of half a dozen regular protesters, none of whom wore masks. A car slowly approached the clinic, the driver looking out his rolled-down window while the passenger kept looking at her phone. An unmasked protester approached the car and stuck his head into the window, coming within inches of the man's face.[36]

"We can help you! You don't have to murder your baby," he implored.

The driver began to roll up his window.

"You'll get coronavirus in there! She'll never come out!"

Cameron-Schwiesow sighed. The pandemic had changed everything, and nothing.

From the Sidewalk to the Suburbs

When Bianca Cameron-Schwiesow's husband was transferred from Germany back to Alabama, she was less than thrilled. She and her husband didn't want to leave Germany, where they had been stationed for several years, but they didn't have much of a choice. She would have to make the best of it. When she arrived in Montgomery in 2018, she decided she wanted to help make Montgomery a more progressive, peaceful community. At a voter registration drive, she met a man who was a clinic escort at Reproductive Health Services. She listened intently as he described how they supported patients, how they tried to maintain a sense of calm and normalcy amid a mass of people shouting at them, how they never engaged with the protesters and always centered the patient and their companions.

That's something that really appeals to me, she thought.[37]

Reproductive Health Services is the only clinic in the southern half of Alabama; the closest clinic to the south, American Family Planning in Pensacola, Florida, is 160 miles away. American Family Planning was formerly known as the Ladies Center, where Dr. Gunn, Dr. Britton, and James Barrett were murdered. While Reproductive Health Services hasn't experienced the level of violence that plagued Pensacola in the 1990s, it has seen its own aggressive and intense antiabortion protests.

In 2015, Operation Save America decided to make Montgomery the site of its annual convention. At the time, Reproductive Health Services was next door to a property that had been vacant for three months. Clinic escorts thought little of it until they read on social media that OSA planned to use it as their protest headquarters.

"The house is so close to the clinic parking lot, if [OSA] were to get the house, they could stand right there on the house property, two feet away and basically at people's front bumpers, and yell at them," Mia Raven, a clinic escort at Reproductive Health Services, explained to *Rolling Stone* in 2016.[38]

Instead, a local group called the Montgomery Area Reproductive Justice Coalition intervened, renting the vacant property from a sympathetic owner, and they have remained there ever since. It became known as the POWER House, and it is the center of clinic escort and other reproductive justice advocacy activities in Montgomery. OSA still protested at the clinic, though they couldn't get as close as they had initially wanted. Hundreds of radical abortion opponents gathered out front, including convicted clinic bomber and eventual anti-mask champion John Brockhoeft.[39] But they all remained behind a police barricade, which blocked off the clinic and the POWER House from protesters.

What was initially a dire threat to the safety of patients became a source of resilience and service, thanks to a supportive landlord and OSA's braggadocio.

By April 1, 2019, Cameron-Schwiesow managed to find a community at the POWER House. Volunteering as a clinic escort was intensely meaningful, and she developed deep friendships with some of her fellow escorts.

That April Fool's Day, she invited a fellow clinic escort over to visit while a maintenance man worked on her house. She walked to the front door to check on his progress when she noticed a card for what she thought was a power washing company. She picked it up and saw instead the image of a man, holding a gun, along with a phone number. Neither she nor her guest had heard the doorbell. She had a gut feeling that something was wrong. She asked the other members of her homeowners' association if they had received a similar flyer. No one else had. She decided to call the number. Upon hearing the voice on the other end of the line, she realized that she knew who it was—it was Daniel French, a frequent protester who had already been charged with destruction of property at the clinic.

The very next day, Alabama state representative Terri Collins introduced the total abortion ban in the Alabama House of Representatives. What felt like an isolated invasion of Cameron-Schwiesow's privacy quickly became a targeted campaign of harassment and intimidation against her, one that coincided with the advancement and ultimate passage of the country's most extreme abortion ban. It wasn't enough to just protest at the clinic anymore. With the possibility of criminalizing abortion entirely,

Alabama antiabortion activists were ready to bring the fight directly to clinic escorts' front doors.

• • •

As April progressed, Alabama moved ever closer toward their total abortion ban. On April 30, 2019, members of the POWER House clinic escort team filed into the Alabama House of Representatives to hear it debate the ban that would eventually be signed into law.

Cameron-Schwiesow was horrified at the potential legislation, knowing that even if it weren't allowed to go into effect, it could increase tension at the clinic and further stigmatize the procedure. She joined other clinic escorts to protest the ban, even dressing up as "handmaids" from Margaret Atwood's *The Handmaid's Tale* at the Alabama State House.[40] But the threat of harassment and violence wasn't an elusive one; it was already at her front door.

While the random card at her front door depicting an armed man wasn't necessarily threatening, that quickly changed. A week later, as her fifteen-year-old son, who has autism, walked toward their neighborhood park, a man in a blue PT Cruiser pulled up alongside him, addressed him by name, and beckoned him over to the car. When her son refused, he shouted, "Did you know your mother's a murderer? Did you know your mom's going to burn in hell for all eternity?"[41]

This wasn't at an abortion clinic or a political rally. This was in a suburban neighborhood. This wasn't even an abortion provider—it was the son of a volunteer clinic escort.

Cameron-Schwiesow called the police, who, she said, failed to take it seriously—they told her to "get another job." She felt isolated and on her own as the harassment continued.

"Daniel [French] followed me," she said. "I do side gigs, like grocery delivery for Walmart, and I remember Daniel following me on numerous occasions, eyeing the cart, looking at me with malice, chasing me and my husband in [our] car, the list goes on and on."

By the time a protester hit Jamie Johnson with a car in Tuscaloosa in early May 2019, Cameron-Schwiesow and her husband were discussing what steps to take to curb the rampant harassment they were experiencing. Just two weeks after Alabama passed a total ban on abortions with no exceptions for rape or incest, Cameron-Schwiesow's family were forced to move to curb the harassment.

• • •

It was just after 5:00 a.m. on May 17, 2019, when Travis Jackson pulled into the parking lot at the POWER House. He went inside, put on a pot of coffee, and grabbed his vest.[42] Cameron-Schwiesow came in soon after, deep circles under her eyes.[43] She hadn't slept much the night before. The last few days had been a blur; ever since the Alabama Senate passed the total abortion ban, it felt like the eyes of the world were on her state. Now that the ban had been signed into law, clinic escorts expected protesters to feel newly emboldened.

They walked outside, all in rainbow vests, well before the sun rose that morning. Jackson headed around back while Cameron-Schwiesow stood near the front door, counting the protesters, counting the news outlets. It was loud, louder than normal. The cry of "You're still going to be a mother, you're just going to be the mother of a dead baby!" pinged off of the POWER House gate. It had barely been an hour before Jackson came running up to her.[44] Jackson, an Iraq War veteran, could usually handle any situation. This must have been something delicate—or really, really bad.

"B, there's a woman here, behind the back door, who keeps

telling me to 'fuck off,'" he explained. "I can't help her. Can you go see what's going on?"

Cameron-Schwiesow walked behind the clinic and found the woman pounding on the back door.

"Excuse me, ma'am, I work here," Cameron-Schwiesow asked. "Can I help you?"

"Fuck off!"

"Ma'am, we don't go in through the back door. Are you a patient?"

"Fuck off! If you can't get the fuck off, I'm going to call the police!"

Cameron-Schwiesow noticed how wide the woman's eyes were, darting from left to right. She didn't know what to do. She motioned for the security officer to come help, and just then, the woman bolted toward the front door. Cameron-Schwiesow took off after her, following her, the woman's backpack bouncing up and down with every move.

The woman grabbed the door, flung it open, and slammed it shut in Cameron-Schwiesow's face. Panicked, Cameron-Schwiesow opened the door, silently praying, *Please god, don't kill anybody. Don't kill anybody, please.*

She opened the door to see the clinic staff huddled around the woman. "She's a patient! It's okay. She's a patient!"

The knot of fear in her stomach immediately fell. She exhaled, then excused herself. She walked over to the POWER House and wept, the adrenaline slowly releasing from her body.

A few hours later, Cameron-Schwiesow saw that woman once again.

"I'm so sorry!" she said between sobs. "I couldn't hear you! I'm so, so sorry."

The woman's cab driver had dropped her off on the sidewalk,

rather than at the parking lot, as was standard. She opened the car door into dozens of angry protesters, calling her a murderer, telling her she would regret this for the rest of her life, warning her that she would never come back out of that building. She had run to the back of the building for relief, to find a way in, to escape the angry mob on the sidewalk. When she saw Jackson and then Cameron-Schwiesow in their rainbow clinic escort vests, she just assumed they were other protesters. She felt cornered and a fight-or-flight reflex kicked in.

"I have children at home," she said. "If I can't have this procedure, I'll die."

Cameron-Schwiesow felt cornered, too, because of the ongoing harassment. Yet this woman was willing to run through a tunnel of terror to get inside. She fought anyone necessary, just to get inside and get an abortion. That was why they were all there. As long as abortion was legal in Alabama, patients like this terrified woman should have someone to support them. They shouldn't be made to feel like wild animals, trapped in a cage of cruelty.

Through the weeks of her own harassment, Cameron-Schwiesow kept showing up to Reproductive Health Services to volunteer. She knew that was why she was being targeted, but she refused to stop. "It's just because I'm a stubborn bitch," she said with a faint laugh. "Nobody has the right to tell a woman what to do. I don't give a shit what you do. You're not going to make me stop supporting people that need this kind of support. You're not going to intimidate me."[45]

• • •

Eric Rudolph wasn't captured until May 31, 2003. He had successfully eluded law enforcement for five years after setting off a deadly bomb at New Woman, All Women Health Clinic in Birmingham, Alabama. A local police officer finally spotted him while he was rummaging through a dumpster in rural North Carolina.[46]

In 2005, he pled guilty to the bombing, accepting a life sentence to avoid the death penalty. During his plea, Rudolph refused to apologize for the bombing and condemned those who opposed abortion but decried his violence as "liars, hypocrites, and cowards." He criticized the piecemeal approach to ending abortion that conservatives at that time seemed to embrace. He cast not just doubt, but condemnation on those who advocated for respectability to end abortion. "They say that pro-life forces are making progress, that eventually *Roe v. Wade* will be overturned, that the culture of life will ultimately win over the majority of Americans and that the horror of abortion will be outlawed," he said, before calling the Republican Party "the modern equivalent to the Pharisaical sect in ancient Judea."[47]

Just seventeen years later, Rudolph's vision of criminalized abortion and mass vigilante violence seemed to bear fruit. Alabama had passed a total abortion ban, and a handful of other states had tried to ban the procedure as early as possible. Hundreds of thousands of Americans had succumbed to COVID-19. Far-right, white nationalist groups were bringing semiautomatic weapons to statehouses in protest of preventive measures to curb the pandemic. By June 2020, as the coronavirus pandemic continued to worsen and outrage over the murder of George Floyd and racist police violence came to the forefront in the United States, Eric Rudolph opened a notebook and scrawled, in slanted capital letters, an appeal to throw out the life sentence he had accepted less than two decades earlier.[48]

For James Silvers, who volunteered as a clinic defender and escort at New Woman, All Women from 1988 to 1991, it was yet another indication of how the Republican Party had aligned itself with far-right extremists. "Things are getting so bad and everything's unraveling," he said. Eric Rudolph saw a moment of opportunity and decided to take it. The crime that had landed him on the FBI's Ten Most Wanted List was being normalized: not just by the Boogaloo Boys screaming at the Ohio Statehouse, but by a president who refused to condemn right-wing militia members like Kyle Rittenhouse, an Illinois teenager who allegedly shot and killed two Black Lives Matter protesters in the summer of 2020.[49]

The clinic that Silvers used to protect with his body, the clinic that Rudolph's shrapnel ripped through, is no more. In the end, it wasn't Rudolph's bomb that ended legal abortion in Birmingham; it was the very political structure he once mocked.

Chapter Six

A Sanctuary State of Mind

I WIGGLED MY FRIGID TOES BACK TO LIFE. TWO PAIRS OF WOOL socks, chemical feet warmers, and thick winter boots were no match for the brutal early-morning New Jersey wind. The sidewalk, narrow enough on its own, had been reduced to a mere plank by the two-foot-high wall of frozen snow lining the curb. I had been a clinic escort for all of ten uneventful minutes, and the only person I approached to walk into the clinic waved me off. Was this all that clinic escort volunteering was, in a liberal state like New Jersey? Just standing here in the freezing cold, ignoring the two silent protesters with CHOOSE LIFE signs?

In January 2014, when I first became a clinic escort, New Jersey was a solidly pro-choice state. With nearly two dozen abortion clinics, it was one of only a handful of states that allowed Medicaid to cover abortion care. When someone approached me and asked if I'd be interested in volunteering as a clinic escort, I honestly didn't know if it was even necessary. How bad could it be in a state like New Jersey, anyway?

That first morning, my initial skepticism was confirmed. Why was I even out here? As I thought of throwing in the towel, a teal van pulled up and parked in a metered spot across the street from the clinic. *Another patient who doesn't need my help*, I thought. In-stead, four men piled out and walked to the back of the van, where a middle-aged man pulled out a stack of giant posters. He handed one to each of the other three, and they walked toward the clinic's front door.

Within minutes, one of them, who was wearing a microphone attached to a personal amp, began screaming toward the door of the clinic.

"God loves that child, but God hates the woman because He hates the doer of iniquity!"

The three other men spread out across the sidewalk, holding their signs aloft, shouting at passersby.

"They're getting paid to murder your baby!"

"There's life in your womb!"

Caught off guard, I stared at them, awash in confusion and frustration.

Our leader, whom we all called "Jane Roe" in honor of *Roe v. Wade*, gestured at me to move a bit farther away from the front door so that I could intercept patients before they reached the growing gauntlet. I waited maybe thirty seconds before I noticed a couple ap-proaching me. The man cradled his companion as they shuffled past the snowbanks. I went up to them and said, as I was trained to do, "Hi, I'm a volunteer with the clinic. I can walk with you, if you'd like." The woman's eyes were glassy—she didn't even acknowledge me. Her companion nodded, and I moved to the other side of the woman. I didn't know what to say after my standard greeting. This woman certainly didn't seem like she wanted to talk, so we walked in silence until a protester, a woman who worked at the antiabortion cri-sis pregnancy center across the street, popped up in front of our faces.

"You don't have to murder your baby," she said in a sweet, cooing voice. "Across the street, we can help you. We can help your baby."

"Please leave us alone," the man said, waving her off.

We kept going, left foot, right foot, left foot, right foot.

"You're such a pretty girl, and your baby will be so pretty, too," she said. "You have other options besides murder!"

"Our baby has spina bifida," boomed the man. "Do you know what that is?"

"Your baby is a gift from God," the protester responded.

"We wanted this baby! We wanted to have this baby and have a family! We are devastated!" The grief and rage in his voice filled the frigid air. I was momentarily stunned. I wanted to scream at this protester, to tell her to get the hell away from these people. But I couldn't. Trained in nonengagement, I knew that I was prohibited from talking to the protesters at all. Instead, I wrapped my right arm around the patient next to me, her body crumpling as she began to sob. Her husband and I shuffled her into the clinic, tears streaming down both of our faces. I later learned that it took an hour for the patient to finally calm down.

I went back out onto the sidewalk in a daze. I looked over at the protester who had so callously disregarded this couple's reality. She looked unfazed as she ran from one snowy side of the street to the other, trying to chase down another couple approaching the clinic. She had no intention of stopping. She had no recognition of the harm she had caused. She just moved right on to the next patient, as the size of the group of men screaming near the front door had doubled in a matter of minutes.

Oh, I realized. This is why I'm here.

That wasn't just my first day as a clinic escort at Metropolitan Medical Associates in Englewood, New Jersey—that was the first patient I ever walked into a clinic. Not every patient has a tragic fetal anomaly or story of sexual assault. Many just don't want to or can't continue their pregnancies. But that day, I saw firsthand the emotional stakes of what happens outside of an abortion clinic, even in a liberal town in a liberal state.

• • •

I had no idea that day that during my six years as a clinic escort, I would watch states outside of New Jersey pass more than four hundred abortion restrictions.[1] By 2020, New Jersey was one of only fourteen states that the Guttmacher Institute classified as "supportive" of abortion rights, while twenty-nine were "hostile" states, with supportive legislation and plentiful abortion clinics becoming the exception rather than the norm. As a result, the abortion rate in New Jersey rose by 9 percent between 2014 and 2017,[2] even though it declined nationally.[3] More people were coming to New Jersey from other more restrictive states to have abortions.

Of course, I didn't realize this at the start of my first shift in January 2014. I knew that more abortion restrictions were enacted from 2011 to 2013 than in the entire previous decade—but that restriction wasn't happening where I was. Technically, that was true: New Jersey and its neighbor New York weren't enacting any restrictions, and both provided Medicaid funding for abortion care.

But blue states haven't been immune to antiabortion protesters; from the very beginning of legal abortion in the United States, clinics in these states have been under attack. Some of the most heinous antiabortion crimes, like the murder of abortion provider Dr. Bart Slepian in his kitchen and the double homicide of clinic workers Shannon Lowey and Leanne Nichols, took place in New York and Massachusetts, two states that have traditionally been very supportive of abortion rights. Operation Rescue began its blockade crusade in Binghamton, New York, and helped fuel national attention with a massive blockade at Cherry Hill Women's Center in Cherry Hill, New Jersey.

On paper, blue states are supportive of abortion rights. Anti-abortion legislators are successfully restricting and banning abortion in Nebraska, Texas, and Missouri, while blue states are more likely to protect abortion rights rather than erode them. The decreasing number of supportive states may end up becoming sanctuary states for legal abortion, but they can also become increasingly easy targets for harassment. If abortion opponents can't hinder access legislatively in states like New York and California, they can do it where they've done it for nearly fifty years: outside the clinics.

One Step Forward, Two Steps Back

It was Valentine's Day 2018, and after more than two years of struggling with infertility, Pearl Brady and her husband were finally pregnant. Brady was back in court, and she was battling the worst nausea she'd ever had in her life. She would try to speak, feel the well of morning sickness bubble up, and have to brace herself to continue. Somehow, she made it through the four days with no spontaneous eruptions.

Brady wasn't in court for work—she was testifying. For the past three years, she had volunteered as a clinic escort at Choices Women's Medical Center in Queens, New York. Now she was on the stand, detailing the years of harassment she witnessed at the clinic.

By 2009, fifteen years after the FACE Act became law, New York City lawmakers realized what many clinic escorts across the country already knew—it wasn't enough. Protesters could still be in close quarters to patients and harass them on a personal, individual level without technically violating the FACE Act by blocking the clinic's entrance. At urban clinics like Choices, which are on public sidewalks and generally lack private parking lots, this allows protesters to be mere feet from the door, able to target each patient. It was clear that more restrictions were needed.

The city's solution was the New York City Access to Reproductive Health Care Facilities Act, commonly known as the NYC Clinic Access Act. The law reinforced elements of the FACE Act and notably created a much wider buffer zone at abortion clinics. Now, any protester who came within fifteen feet of a clinic's entrance would be in violation of city law and could be prosecuted. New York City abortion clinics like Choices suddenly had a new tool to reduce harassment and improve patient security.[4]

As a former clinic escort at a Planned Parenthood in Manhattan, Brady knew the law. By the time she began volunteering at Choices, the clinic had posted printed copies of the New York City buffer zone law and the FACE Act in their windows.

When Becca Ballenger arrived at Choices at 6:30 a.m. on her first Saturday as a volunteer in 2015, she was surprised to find a group of protesters already gathered outside the clinic. Protesters started showing up to Choices as early as 6:00 a.m. to stake out their positions.[5] Ballenger quickly realized that what was legal and what was tolerated were two different things. "The fifteen-foot buffer zone sounds *so nice*," said Ballenger. "It basically doesn't exist, in reality. [On my first day] I was shocked by how close [the protesters] would get."[6]

That's because they could, and they knew they could. The New York City police department didn't seem to take it seriously, something Ballenger saw the first time the police were ever called to Choices during her shift. "There was one community affairs officer—he would typically be the one [who] would come [in response to a complaint]," she said. "He would always go right to the pastor of the church and shake his hand, give him a hug, talk to him.

And then, he'd come over to [the clinic escorts] and say 'What are you doing to restrict their First Amendment rights today?' That was one the first things he said to me."[7]

It was the protesters, not the staff or even the police, who established the dynamic and the tone outside Choices. Without any meaningful enforcement, they continued to escalate their behavior.

One frequent protest group, the Church @ the Rock, would bring people with disabilities to the clinic to protest, a tactic I heard about from several clinic escort groups across the country. Some would be given gory signs to hold, standing quietly off to the side. But some were much more aggressive, walking right up to patients and even screaming at them. "They were actually instructed [by Church @ the Rock leaders] to be most aggressive toward patients because their disability makes intervention more delicate for the patient and for the escorts," explained Moira Donegan, another clinic escort at Choices. Protesters were almost goading clinic escorts and patients into a confrontation, seemingly exploiting people with disabilities to do their bidding.

Perhaps not surprisingly, abortion opponents have been criticized before for using people with disabilities as pawns. In response to a proposed "disability abortion ban" in Florida, Robyn Powell, a professor who studies the intersection of disability and abortion rights (and has arthrogryposis, which leaves her with limited use of her arms and legs), slammed the bill as "using disability as a justification to take abortion rights away," claiming it would hurt those who were already the most vulnerable, rather than support people with disabilities. Olivia Babis, a senior public policy analyst at Disability Rights Florida and herself a woman with a disability, asked for special accommodations by the Florida House of Representatives, due to her disability, to be able to testify regarding the bill. Her request was denied.[8]

For Ballenger, the most emblematic moment of the worsening situation came during a Saturday in the summer of 2016. Ballenger and another clinic escort were walking with a patient and her companion, neither of whom spoke English. As they approached the clinic, "a protester came so close behind a patient that they stepped on her flip-flop and broke [it]." The woman stopped, unsure of what to do with a broken shoe and another ten steps to the clinic entrance. She was forced to walk on a New York City sidewalk with only one shoe because a protester had willingly violated the law. "It was just so chaotic and horrible and difficult to communicate," Ballenger said. "That kind of thing was starting to happen a lot more, this total chaos close to the door."[9]

Clinic escorts at Choices were used to this. They had already learned how to navigate around the protesters standing in front of the door, screaming nonstop for hours and practically walking on top of anyone approaching the clinic, simply to support people who needed to get inside. They knew calling the police was basically a nonstarter—not only would they most likely refuse to enforce the buffer zone, but Ballenger would watch some NYPD officers fist-bump some of the protesters in support. This was just the way it was going to have to be in Queens, Choices clinic escorts reasoned. Abortion was legal, but harassment was apparently acceptable.

On June 20, 2017, that changed. Eric Schneiderman, then the New York attorney general, announced a federal lawsuit against the antiabortion protesters at Choices. The lawsuit included a preliminary injunction that barred protesters from any unlawful conduct and established a sixteen-foot buffer zone. While only nominally larger than the city's existing fifteen-foot buffer zone, an accompanying lawsuit from the highest law enforcement officer in the state could make it less likely that protesters would violate that barrier. "The tactics used to harass and menace Choices' patients,

families, volunteers, and staff are not only horrifying—they're illegal," Attorney General Schneiderman said in a press release. "The
law guarantees women the right to control their own bodies and
access the reproductive health care they need, without obstruction.
We'll do what it takes to protect those rights for women across
New York."[10]

For the first time in years, it seemed like someone in power was
taking the claims of harassment seriously that Choices clinic escorts,
staff, and patients had been making for years. "I was excited," Ballenger recalled. "I was so hopeful."[11]

When Pearl Brady ultimately took the stand in 2018, she was
determined to muscle through morning sickness to share all that
she had seen and experienced—not just for her, but for her fellow
clinic escorts, for the staff, and for every patient who'd been forced to
endure harassment and humiliation. It felt like the protesters might
finally be forced to take responsibility for their unlawful behavior.
Perhaps the atmosphere outside Choices could begin to resemble
what it should have always been—just another health-care facility.

• • •

Sitting in the middle of a city council meeting on March 19, 2014,
surrounded by yellow vests on one side and bloody fetus signs on the
other, it finally dawned on Ashley Gray what a whirlwind the last six
months of her life had become.

In the fall of 2013, Gray saw an article in a local New Jersey
paper about the escalating protests outside Metropolitan Medical Associates. A group of "street preachers"—all of whom were men—
were protesting there, and the dynamics outside the clinic became
tenuous, sometimes verging on violence. Gray lived in New York
then, but MMA wasn't far from where she grew up. Shocked and

horrified, she called the clinic and asked if they needed volunteers or if she could join their clinic escort team.

"We don't have one of those," the MMA staff member responded. "But another woman actually called and asked the same thing just a few hours ago. If you two want to talk, I can give you her number."

Gray said yes and called the woman, another New Yorker who called herself "Jane Roe." They immediately connected. By the end of the phone call, they decided to create a clinic escort team at MMA, the team I ended up joining just a few months later.[12]

Neither Gray nor "Roe" had ever volunteered as a clinic escort before. Longtime leaders like Benita Ulisano of Chicago offered advice, training materials, and even free vests. They started reaching out to the people in their lives—friends, family members, people in their community who might be willing to join them in this new endeavor.

The first few times they walked out onto the sidewalk, there were only three of them, sometimes up against dozens of protesters. Gray and "Roe" quickly noticed that even though there were a significant number of protesters, they didn't all seem to know each other. Some, members of a Korean Catholic community, simply stood across the street, holding a framed picture of Jesus Christ while quietly praying. They never seemed to bother anyone or interfere with patients' access in any way.

Then there were the women who worked at the antiabortion crisis pregnancy center across the street. Some of them were quiet, simply holding signs and trying to politely hand out literature to anyone who walked past. But some were pushier and downright nasty. One, who we later dubbed "The Runner" because she would run for blocks after people who walked in and out of the clinic, would stand as close to a patient as possible, sometimes cutting off their path to the door. She walked backward, so her face was in the patient's face the entire time, muttering in a sickly sweet voice about how abortion was murder and a tragedy, that God gave you this baby and you should be grateful, all the way to the door of the clinic. She would inevitably be waiting to harass patients after their abortion, following them all the way to their car, telling them to pray for forgiveness and repent for their sins. She could reduce any patient to tears with her utter refusal to leave people alone and let them be.

By far the worst was the group Gray read about in the local newspaper, the men from a fundamentalist church called the Bread of Life, who fashioned themselves as "street preachers." This group, led by fundamentalist Joseph LoSardo, took protesting to an entirely new level.[13] While one of them would "street preach" by yelling through a megaphone about the horrors of abortion and the evil jezebels who went into the clinic to kill their babies, the others would spread out to various points on the sidewalk so they could intercept anyone approaching the clinic. Some held up gruesome, doctored pictures of bloody fetuses or a crudely drawn BABIES ARE MURDERED HERE sign with fake blood splattered on it. They would quite literally scream at people who walked up to the clinic, calling them murderers, sinners, devils. The Bread of Life protesters were willing to get much more physical than the other groups—they would target men who accompanied women into the clinic, pointing in their faces, telling them to be a man, to not let this jezebel murder their baby. They seemed to revel in their own ability to inflict suffering on others.

By the time I attended my training session in early January 2014, Gray and "Roe" knew the ins and outs of each of these groups and had already had their own challenges in trying to walk patients past the growing anarchy outside the clinic. They warned us that the men from the Bread of Life Church were furious that the clinic now had escorts, and they would often turn their ire on those of us in vests.

That was a good thing, they explained. That meant they weren't targeting patients. But it also meant that we would have to be calm and composed in the face of direct and often deeply personal cruelty. We should be prepared to be called "fat," "stupid," "ugly," "evil," "bloodthirsty," or any other horrible adjective we could think of, Gray explained. They had already heard their fair share. No matter what they said, we were not to engage with the protesters. Our focus was to remain on the patient, to make sure that they could walk into the clinic as safely and as unimpeded as possible. We weren't there for the protesters—we were there to let the patients know that they weren't alone, that they had support, that they deserved to feel safe.

For the first three months of 2014, I was at the clinic every single weekend; we all were. There simply weren't enough of us to be able to split up into smaller teams. Normally, two clinic escorts would walk with a patient and companion, one on either side, using our outstretched arms to keep protesters from jumping up at their sides. But on days when the Bread of Life protesters brought in protesters from out of state, the numbers on the sidewalk would swell, and we'd adjust our tactics. Four of us would form a bubble around patients and companions, one in the front, one in the back, and two on the sides. We would move as a unit, as quickly as we could, desperately trying to get to the door while keeping the patient safe and secure with our bodies as shields.

I learned how to read patients' body language, how to gauge if they needed someone to crack a joke or if they wanted to walk in silence. Some would ask me, "Why are they doing this?" afraid that the protesters would hurt them. A few eschewed my offer and walked right past the group—some with middle fingers up, defiantly entering the clinic. But most just wanted privacy, anonymity. They wanted to be able to walk into this health-care facility like they would any other—nameless, faceless, unrecognized—and go about their day. When they were faced with the reality of strangers screaming at them, filming them with cell phones, trying to block their path on the sidewalk, many were confused and apprehensive. Even though they had been told by the clinic that protesters would be there and they should look for the "people in the vests," most patients didn't realize they needed a clinic escort until that moment.

Englewood is right across the George Washington Bridge from New York City, and that proximity is reflected in its decidedly liberal political leaning.[14] The local news coverage that helped spur the creation of my clinic escort team also fueled outrage from Englewood citizens and City Councilmember Lynne Algrant, herself a former clinic escort. Before I joined the fledgling team in January 2014, there were only three volunteers out front, including Gray and "Roe." On one of their first few days, Councilmember Algrant pulled up in front of the clinic, handed Gray a business card, and said, "I'm on the City Council. If you have any problems, please call me."[15]

That business card marked the beginning of a monthslong collaborative relationship. After every Saturday morning shift at the clinic, Gray and "Roe" filed formal reports with the clinic's lawyer, the city council, and the Englewood chief of police, detailing the number of protesters at our clinic and the range of their behavior, including some that was clearly unlawful. Every week, our small team kept showing up, filming encounters on our phones, and taking pictures of every infraction we saw. Local advocates joined the chorus, and soon the city council started exploring legislative means to abate the harassment at MMA, ultimately considering an eight-foot buffer zone at the city's abortion clinics. That's what led Gray to this moment in March 2014, seated in the Englewood City Council meeting.

Our entire team, about two dozen people at that point, attended the meeting, clad in our bright yellow vests. There were protesters, too, but they were significantly outnumbered by the strong show of support for us and the clinic by the community. One after another, Englewood residents rose to testify about the harassment they had seen outside MMA, how it was counter to the city's values, and why an eight-foot buffer zone was the least the city could do to try to curb it.

As the meeting progressed, our anxiety began to build. It seemed possible, even likely, that the city council would pass the buffer zone. But after an antiabortion lawyer named Edward Gilhooly testified that he would immediately file suit if the city did enact a buffer zone, I felt less certain about the outcome.[16] Everyone knew that the Supreme Court was currently weighing the constitutionality of a Massachusetts law that mandated a thirty-five-foot buffer zone (which would be struck down later that year).[17] What if Englewood was too afraid to take the risk?

I sat next to my fellow clinic escort Kaye Toal, both of us filled with nervous energy. In front of me were six of my fellow volunteers. We all collectively gripped hands as the city council prepared to vote on the measure. My chest thumped and my gut tightened—this was it. Councilmember Michael Cohen grabbed the thin microphone in front of his seat, straightening his spine as he pulled it toward him. "In Englewood, we don't follow—we lead."

Down the row, Gray looked over at us, tears gathering in her eyes. None of us would know each other if Gray hadn't read that article and decided to do something about harassment at the clinic. None of this would be happening. There would be no buffer zone proposal. There would be no clinic escort team. There would be no momentum to improve the safety and security of abortion patients in this small city. She felt the weight of that accomplishment and responsibility. As the air filled with "Ayes," she finally felt a release.

"The measure is adopted!"

Gray burst into tears.[18] We clapped and shouted. Somehow, we had done it! We had created a real change for MMA and its patients. It wasn't enough, we knew. Eight feet is hardly anything. But it was something. It was real, and we felt that it was just the start. This was a liberal town in a liberal state, and we had real momentum, we thought.

That victory would be short-lived; the legal challenge from abortion opponents was coming. As is so often the case in abortion rights, it would be one step forward, two steps back.

• • •

When a new class of New York state legislators was sworn in on January 10, 2019, it had some new faces. While the country grappled with the nomination of accused sexual assailant Brett Kavanaugh to the Supreme Court, and what his appointment could mean for the future of *Roe v. Wade*, candidates in the blue state of New York took up that fight as their own. Newly elected state senators like Zellnor Myrie had pushed the state senate, long dominated by Democrats but with a few conservative holdouts, further to the left, with many embracing reproductive rights as part of their plank in the fall of 2018.

One of their first priorities upon inauguration was shoring up the state's abortion statute. When New York legalized abortion in 1970, its law wasn't as expansive as *Roe v. Wade* dictated three years later. The new federal ruling simply overrode the state law, and abortion was legal up to twenty-four weeks. Modifying the state law wasn't a priority—it wasn't necessary as long as abortion was protected by federal law. But now that the Supreme Court had tilted against abortion rights, the end of *Roe v. Wade* seemed more plausible. If that happened, New York's outdated abortion statute would take over, rendering the state more restrictive than it had been for nearly fifty years under *Roe*.

The solution was the Reproductive Health Act (RHA), which amended the state's public health law by removing outdated provisions, like abortion's inclusion in the criminal code, and enshrining abortion's legality up to twenty-four weeks of pregnancy, and after that point if the health or life of the pregnant person is in danger.[19] There was nothing new or radical about the RHA—it simply brought New York's state law in line with *Roe v. Wade*. But it signaled to the rest of the country that New York would remain the abortion rights leader it had been for nearly half a century.

When New York governor Andrew Cuomo signed the RHA into law on January 22, 2019, the forty-sixth anniversary of the *Roe* decision, he explained why this legislation was important to more than just New Yorkers. "With the signing of this bill, we are sending a clear message that whatever happens in Washington, women in New York will always have the fundamental right to control their own body."[20]

It was a victory for abortion rights. After years of restrictions, it signaled that not every state was hostile to legal abortion. But the RHA only ensured that abortion would remain legal—it didn't address the pervasive, decades-long problem of antiabortion harassment. That's what the NYC Clinic Access Law was supposed to do, and that's what the federal lawsuit against the protesters at Choices was meant to help establish. Instead, clinic escorts were left to keep harassment at bay. Legally, patients are protected. In reality, their experience depends on the number of protesters that day, and the number of vests.

• • •

As the coronavirus pandemic ravaged the United States throughout 2020, "six feet" took on a new meaning. In order to prevent the transmission of COVID-19, everyone was encouraged to remain at least six feet away from each other—in other words, to practice social distancing. In the age of a pandemic, when someone violates that barrier and comes closer to you, particularly if they are unmasked, it feels like a gross violation and intrusion.

Now, imagine that unmasked person coming within six feet of you—even ten feet—as you walk into a health-care clinic, and they're screaming at you. You can see the spit flying out of their mouth. You can feel the air become saturated with their salivary particles. You don't know what else they might do. You just want to get inside.

Six feet isn't much, but that distance can provide a sense of security and safety. It's not a guarantee. It's just one less stressor in an already stressful situation.

This is exactly what a buffer zone does—it simply keeps protesters from getting right up in the faces of people entering an abortion clinic. In the fall of 2014, when the eight-foot buffer zone ordinance finally went into effect, the front door of the New Jersey clinic where I volunteered no longer felt like a war zone. Protesters were free to approach patients and even walk with them, but not once they reached that safety zone at the door. Eight feet. It's barely larger than the six feet of socially distanced propriety our public health now demands. But it made a noticeable difference in the atmosphere at the clinic, and it provided solace for patients.

"We just have to get to that yellow line," I started saying to patients. "Once we're in there, they can't come near you. Just get to that yellow line."

Our entire model shifted. Now that protesters couldn't be within eight feet of the entrance, we didn't have to get there as the sun rose to ensure that we beat them to the positions on either side of the front door. Instead, we were able to shrink our weekly team by half, putting one person at the door and a handful of other escorts to walk patients through the ever-present protesters into the buffer zone. Patients relaxed, knowing that there was a safe zone for them. Protesters could still talk to them and engage with them, but they couldn't block a patient's way or physically intimidate them right at the door. It was still chaotic, but it was progress.

It was no surprise when one of the protesters eventually filed a lawsuit against the buffer zone, claiming that it interfered with her First Amendment rights. Antiabortion attorney Edward Gilhooly had said as much in the city council meeting, and we knew it wasn't an idle threat. But we were optimistic. Even though Massachusetts's thirty-five-foot buffer zone had recently been ruled unconstitutional by the Supreme Court in *McCullen v. Coakley*, our buffer zone was much smaller, and it applied to all health-care facilities in the city, not just abortion clinics.[21] It was actually written with the then-pending Supreme Court case in mind, designed to hold up to inevitable legal challenges.

The law giveth, and the law taketh away.

On November 16, 2017, Gray let me know that a district court judge had struck down Englewood's buffer zone, ruling it a violation of the protester's right to free speech. Two days later, our team was back at the clinic, except this time, protesters didn't have to stay eight feet away. They could get as close to the door and to patients as they wanted, and we couldn't stop them.

At first, the Bread of Life protesters didn't realize that the buffer zone had been struck down. But as soon as they did, they planted themselves directly in front of the door. One shift, I positioned myself at the door, and a protester, who was at least a foot taller than me, stood so close to me that I could feel his breath on my neck. He jammed his elbow in and out of my back, goading me to respond. I stood my ground, moving my body around his to open the door when other escorts walked up with patients.

"Jezebel," he muttered to me. "Horrible, wicked woman."

I noticed another patient approaching the door. I swiveled my body around the protester to block him from getting in her face as she walked by. As she approached the door, I swiveled back across him to open it.

"There you go," I said as I closed the door behind her. I looked the protester in the eye, my lips curling into a defiant smile. "They can't bother you in there!"

• • •

Becca Ballenger sat in the Brooklyn courthouse, shifting in her seat. She wasn't testifying in the case against Choices Women's Medical Center protesters, but she wanted to support Pearl Brady and others who were. She wanted to show up for Choices and for their patients. She wanted to be in the room where it happened.

Brady was right in the middle of that "it" as one of the prosecution's key witnesses against the protesters. For four days, she endured brutal morning sickness to speak her truth about what really happened outside Choices. As a result of the trial, the protesters finally learned her real name, and they began taunting her outside the courtroom. They plastered her name and image across antiabortion blogs and news sites. Her social media accounts and inboxes were filled with bile and cruelty. She even had to alert HR at her workplace to the possibility of targeted harassment there. By the fourth and final day of testimony, she was exhausted. "It was one of the hardest things I've ever done in my life," she said. "Having to be in the same room as the protesters, all day for four days, was really hard."[22]

At the beginning, Ballenger came as often as she could. But as the trial dragged on, a knot of discomfort began to grow in her stomach. It seemed to her that Judge Carol Bagley Amon wasn't particularly swayed by the mountains of evidence that Choices clinic escorts thought they had provided. Ballenger decided not to come for the final day of Brady's testimony. "By the end, I was pretty disheartened. It seemed very clear me how it was going to fall out by the end and I just couldn't bear it anymore."[23]

Five months later, well into her third trimester, Brady was trying to stay cool on a warm summer day when she received the news. Judge Amon had ruled against them, writing that the attorney general's office had "failed to show" that any of the thirteen defendants "had the intent to harass, annoy, or alarm" patients at the clinic.[24]

Not only that, but Judge Amon criticized some of the witnesses for exaggerating claims of harassment and impropriety and dismissed the questionnaires in which patients described the treatment they experienced at the hands of those protesters as "hearsay."

She understood that you didn't always win, that sometimes the luck of the draw wasn't on your side. But she was also a clinic escort, and a witness in this case. She took the ruling personally.

"It was very upsetting to me that the judge essentially disregarded all of the clinic escort testimony. She pretty much blanket disregarded all of it . . . It seemed to me like we didn't really have a chance, when I read the decision, because there were certain sweeping decisions that were made that didn't make sense to me. It was really upsetting because we had worked really hard and I felt like the evidence that we had was extremely, extremely strong. All of the video that we had. I was really disappointed."[25]

The very next day, a Saturday morning, the protesters were back at Choices. The law hadn't changed; it was still technically illegal in New York City for them to be within fifteen feet of the clinic. But the law had failed abortion patients yet again. The police weren't going to enforce the law. The judiciary wasn't going to enforce it. The only people who were going to protect the patients were the same people who had been protecting them for years—clinic escorts.

"Being a body on the sidewalk, walking with someone, smiling at someone—one little moment actually makes a difference," Ballenger said about continuing to volunteer at Choices. "That feels really important to me. I'm disillusioned [with] the idea that we can change anything legally right now in this climate at Choices, but I do feel like . . . if somebody smiles at me or if I tell [someone] that their shoes are cute and they don't see a sign with a bloody fetus, then that's one little thing that I did that made it a little bit better. There's not a whole lot that a person on their own can do that actually feels like you're doing something at all, and this is something."[26]

The Reality of a "Regional Hub"

As she crossed the river from Missouri to Illinois one morning in September 2020, Robin Frisella watched the sun rise ahead of her. She recalled the first time she made this drive eight years ago, the determination she felt, the anxiety that fluttered in her stomach. It was a quick drive—barely fifteen minutes start to finish, but it felt much longer in 2012. Now, dozens of trips later, it felt like second nature.

In 2012, Frisella found out she was pregnant, and she knew she didn't want to be. She swiftly and assuredly decided to have an abortion. The St. Louis resident knew she had very few options if she wanted to stay in-state for an abortion—at that point, there were only two clinics left in Missouri, both run by Planned Parenthood.[27] Instead, she decided to do the next best thing and drive across the river to Illinois for an abortion.

Granite City, Illinois, isn't known for much. It's a small post-industrial town with just under thirty thousand residents.[28] But since 1974, it has been home to an enduring institution, one that now plays host to an ever-increasing number of out-of-staters in need: the Hope Clinic for Women.

"I wasn't struggling with the decision," Frisella recalled. "I felt confident. But as I was driving in to the clinic . . . I knew to expect protesters." She was right. Frisella's appointment was on a week-day, which meant that, although there were fewer protesters, there weren't any clinic escorts, who only came on Saturday mornings. She parked her car in the lot and exhaled. She knew she was going to have to walk to the door of the clinic, past the taunts of "Murderer!" and the gory fetus signs, by herself. She was nervous, but resolute. She needed an abortion, and she was going to get one.

Walking through the protesters by herself motivated Frisella. She didn't want anyone else to have to face what she did. That's why, in September 2020, she was once again in her car on the Poplar Street Bridge, driving across the Mississippi River to Illinois. She wasn't going to get an abortion—she was volunteering as a clinic escort.[29]

• • •

In the summer of 2019, just months after New York paved the way, Illinois passed its own Reproductive Health Act, shoring up the state's abortion code and ensuring that it would remain a safe place for safe, legal abortion, regardless of what happened with the Supreme Court.[30]

Illinois is the most reliably Democratic state in the Midwest. Home to the third most populous city in the nation, Chicago, it hasn't gone "red" in a presidential election since 1988.[31] What makes Illinois all the more unique is its location. It neighbors some of the most reliably conservative states in the Midwest, if not the country. Five states border Illinois—Indiana, Wisconsin, Iowa, Kentucky, and Missouri—all of which went for Trump in 2016,[32] four of which went for him again in 2020.[33] Two of those states, Missouri and Kentucky, had only one abortion clinic left before *Dobbs* in June 2022. Illinois also has far fewer restrictions on abortion than Missouri and Indiana, which both have mandatory waiting periods in effect. If patients are able to drive to Illinois, they won't be subjected to more than one trip to the clinic. They can just go, get a safe and legal abortion, and leave.

Missouri's proximity to Illinois is largely why Robin Frisella decided to have an abortion there, rather than at home in St. Louis, and it's why, as abortion has become more restricted across the Midwest, a greater number of patients are following her example.[34]

Illinois, like New York, has taken concrete legal steps to protect abortion rights in the state. As its neighbors move in the opposite direction, the state has become not only a leader, but a loner in the Midwest. Illinois is now a regional hub for abortion care, and if *Roe v. Wade* ever falls, it will likely be one of a few states in the area with reliable access, if not the only one. The state is now a sanctuary for abortion. Legally, it's a protective sphere.

This puts tremendous pressure on the clinics in Illinois, and on the volunteers who serve them. "While I'm glad that Illinois can serve as a bastion and can be a place for resources, I do get concerned about our resources being overwhelmed and just the ability of people to access them," said Amanda Ehrhardt, a clinic escort at Family Planning Associates in Chicago. "You're talking about, in some cases, people coming from low-income situations in which taking a day off work, or getting a hotel room, or getting a bus ticket, that might be out of their means."[35]

Of course, patients aren't the only ones who are traveling farther to get to an abortion clinic. Antiabortion protesters are traveling, too. They know that clinics in Illinois are attracting more patients. If they can't end abortion in sanctuary states like Illinois, they can at least make getting one as unpleasant as possible.

• • •

When Alison Dreith was growing up, Granite City had already passed its heyday. Dreith, a native of Madison County, which includes Granite City, loved to hear stories from her grandparents about going dancing every weekend in the "East St. Louis" community, as it was known. But now, Granite City, like many cities and towns in the region, is an economically stagnant shell of its former self. It's also bleeding residents—the most recent census recorded a 5.62 percent decline in population since 2010.[36]

But one place in Granite City is attracting more people lately, and not just from neighboring Missouri. Cars with license plates from Kentucky, Ohio, and even Virginia have filled the parking lot of Hope Clinic for Women. What Robin Frisella did to access abortion care in 2012 has become standard for pregnant people across the Midwest, and even beyond. Now that Illinois is one of the only states that has protected abortion rights within its borders, Hope Clinic has become a go-to destination for legal abortion care.

It's also home to increasingly aggressive antiabortion protesters. That's why, particularly on weekends, Hope Clinic has an active, dedicated clinic escort team. What Robin Frisella experienced as a weekday abortion patient in 2012 pales in comparison to what the clinic has experienced in more recent years. Motivated by Missouri's dwindling number of abortion providers and emboldened by restrictive legislation across the country, abortion opponents have zeroed in on Hope Clinic.

In early 2016, Justine Colom also came from Missouri to Hope Clinic, but for a very different reason—she wanted to help. Colom was raised to be "super pro-life" in a staunchly Catholic house. As a child, she seemed destined to join those with signs and bullhorns outside Hope Clinic. But in her early twenties, she had a change of heart and came to support abortion rights. She thought it was important, but didn't feel compelled to get involved until a decade later, as her home state of Missouri was left with a single abortion clinic. She decided to become a clinic escort. The St. Louis Planned Parenthood was closer, but Hope Clinic was just across the river. Plus, she knew the need was greater. At the Planned Parenthood, patients could pull into a parking lot free from protesters. At Hope, once the few spots in the small private parking lot fill up, patients have to park in a public lot, and protesters can get as close as they want.[37]

A patient having someone on their side, who is there to support them and provide a buffer from the hostility, is always good. When they've had to travel hundreds of miles on an already stressful morning? It can be essential.

Dreith doesn't live in her home county anymore, but she does remain intimately involved: she's the communications director for Hope Clinic, and she has watched as the climate outside her clinic has grown increasingly tense over the past few years. "Their language has changed dramatically," she said. "It's disgusting."[38]

Granite City's population is mostly white, as are most of the protesters.[39] But Hope Clinic's patients are much more racially diverse. Many Black patients and patients of color come across the river from Missouri because they know that Hope Clinic is one of the only reliable places that they can go to access care. After Ferguson, Missouri, when police officer Darren Wilson killed unarmed Black teenager Mike Brown and the Black Lives Matter movement began in 2014, the majority-white protesters outside Hope Clinic began to use more explicitly racialized and racist language. Mariceli Algeria, clinic support coordinator for NARAL Missouri and a clinic escort at Hope Clinic, said the protesters reserve their harshest rhetoric for Black patients and companions.

"Hey man, don't you want to teach your baby how to sag his pants like you do?"

"Don't you want to teach your baby how to play basketball?"

"Don't you think that Black lives matter? These white [clinic escorts] are marching you in here to murder your Black baby because *they're* racist."[40]

No one can erase the barbarity of racist comments. All that clinic escorts can do is hope to serve as a mitigating factor in an otherwise deeply unpleasant and perhaps even traumatizing interaction and help defuse the tension.

May 11, 2019, the day before Mother's Day, was an abnormally cold day in Granite City.[41] Colom arrived bright and early at Hope Clinic for her morning shift, ready for the chill and the busy day ahead. After three years of volunteering, she knew what to expect. The protests were bigger and more organized around 40 Days for Life and days like Mother's Day and Father's Day. Today was going to be tough, she figured.

Sure enough, within half an hour, the public parking lot next to Hope Clinic was filled with dozens of protesters. The clinic's private parking lot was already full, which meant that patients had nowhere else to go but right into the belly of the beast. Colom approached a car in the lot. Inside were two women, one young, one older. Colom thought it was likely a mother and daughter. She introduced herself: "Hi, I'm a volunteer with the clinic. I can walk with you, if you'd like."

The two women nodded, and Colom began to walk with them, holding her arm out by her side to try to provide a bit more of a buffer.

"You're going to be murdering your dead grandbaby!"

"Aren't you two going to have a great Mother's Day, thinking about the dead baby you could have had?"[42]

Colom winced. The younger woman bowed her head as tears filled her eyes. Her mother whipped around, her eyes filled with anger and horror. She looked at the man who was screaming this invective at her and her daughter. Colom knew what he was trying to do—he wanted to get under their skin. He wanted to start a fight. She quietly said, "Just keep walking. We're almost there."

Finally, they reached the door. As they began to walk inside, they heard, "Tomorrow's Mother's Day, and all you're going to be thinking about is your dead baby that you murdered!"

Colom closed the door with a flourish. She couldn't ease the sting of the cruelty they experienced, but at least they were inside. They were going to be okay. They had made it. Colom made her way back to the public parking lot.

A few minutes later, a car pulled up with a woman in the passenger's seat and two children in the back. As the woman opened her door, Colom greeted her. The woman didn't respond. She had deep bags under eyes. The same protester that harassed the mother and daughter came up, and Colom tried to put her body between them.

"Did you tell your kids that you're here to murder their little brother or sister?" he taunted.

Colom glanced at the car's license plate. Oklahoma.

She glanced back at the woman, who met her gaze. They began to walk, slowly, silently, toward the clinic. This woman had already driven hundreds of miles that morning so that she could have an abortion. They were getting in the door.

• • •

Chicago may be in the same state as Granite City, but the two are divided by more than just three hundred miles—they're entirely different worlds. Fewer than thirty thousand people live in Granite City; 2.6 million people call Chicago home.[43] Fifty-five percent of Madison County's voters went for Donald Trump in 2020, while Chicago's Cook County went heavily for Joe Biden, nearly three in four voters.[44] Granite City has one abortion clinic; Chicago, one of the few remaining cities with numerous options for abortion care, has fifteen,[45] and that's just in the city proper.

Chicago's abundance of abortion clinics makes up for the dearth of access in the rest of the state. While Hope Clinic for Women is now joined by a brand new state-of-the-art Planned Parenthood facility in neighboring Fairview Heights, most of the clinics in the state are located in the Chicago metropolitan area.[46] As neighboring states like Indiana and Wisconsin have restricted abortion, and even for southern Illinoisans who would rather trek to the big city than down to the only clinic in Missouri, Chicago has become the go-to destination.

Jay Griffin watched that happen over their six years as a clinic escort (Griffin identifies as nonbinary and uses they/them pronouns). Griffin started out at a clinic on the North Side of Chicago, which had a large, private space outside the clinic that meant fewer protesters and a relative calm. Chicago has an eight-foot bubble zone, which requires protesters to remain eight feet away from people approaching an abortion clinic.[47] In Griffin's experience, the protesters generally abided by it. "I was stationed there with a very experienced escort, who helped me out and gave me the lay of the land," they said. "My first few times out were boring more than anything else. That place didn't attract a lot of attention on the weekdays."[48]

Griffin soon switched to Family Planning Associates (FPA) on Washington Street, right in the heart of downtown Chicago, the main clinic at which longtime clinic escort Benita Ulisano volunteers. The atmosphere at FPA was completely different from what Griffin had seen previously. There was very little private space outside the clinic, allowing protesters more access to patients. To Griffin, Chicago's bubble zone did not seem to exist here like it did at the other clinic. "[Protesters] were actually approaching the patients and trying to talk to them and hand them literature," Griffin said. "That took me aback."[49]

"You don't need a big group of protesters to do damage," Ulisano explained. "We could be out there and have one aggressive protester who just says the most vile shit to someone and that will make them cry . . . That's the thing—one of them out there is too many."[50]

As the 2010s progressed, Griffin and Ulisano both noticed an escalation among protesters at FPA. There wasn't a significant increase in their numbers, but their behavior changed. They became more emboldened, more targeted on individual patients, more pointed in their cruelty. After Donald Trump won the presidential election in 2016, a mix of corrosive political bile and personalized harassment made it even more difficult for clinic escorts to mitigate the tension.

When I asked if there was a particular patient that they recalled, Griffin didn't hesitate. A girl, likely still in high school, according to Griffin's estimation, came to FPA one day in 2018. She was with an older man, who had wrapped his arm around her in a defensive posture. Griffin approached them and began to escort them to clinic, matching the duo's pace and speaking in a calm, steady tone. "The door is over there," Griffin said. "We're almost there."

As soon as they began to approach the clinic, a group of protesters swooped in. "The antis started addressing him as though he was the one who had gotten her pregnant."[51]

The man jerked his head. "What the hell is wrong with you? That's my daughter!"

"Don't let your daughter murder your grandbaby!"

One of the protesters tried to hand an antiabortion pamphlet to the young girl, whose eyes were squeezed shut.

"Get the hell away from my daughter right now!"

Griffin knew that the protesters had this girl's father right where they wanted him—on the verge of physically assaulting them. That would allow the protesters to call the police, file a report, and position themselves as victims rather than perpetrators of harm. Griffin felt that the clinic escorts needed to step in to avoid a confrontation.

"It took three of us for that," Griffin remembered. A clinic escort locked arms with the young girl and walked her into the clinic. Griffin and another volunteer positioned themselves on either side of her father, attempting to "talk him down and convince him that it wasn't worth assaulting [the protesters]."

The girl's father didn't hit anyone that day. The protesters escaped yet another encounter unscathed, unsuccessful in goading him into a physical confrontation, and Griffin believes that clinic escorts are the reason.

"It would have escalated," Griffin said. "I can very easily see a version of that day that ends with him in the back of the squad car while his daughter is going in for a pretty intense medical procedure."[52]

A few hours later, that man opened the clinic door for his daughter, gently cradling her as she stepped out of the clinic. The protesters were long gone, and so were the clinic escorts. She looked in front of her and saw what she should have seen hours before—nothing.

• • •

It's a point of pride for Benita Ulisano that her hometown is a port in a storm of restriction to abortion access. No matter what happens with national abortion politics, even if *Roe v. Wade* is ultimately overturned, she knows that Illinois will continue to be a leader. She also knows that passing laws is only part of the struggle—enforcing them is another. Even more challenging is creating a cultural shift around this divisive issue, one that reverberates beyond the borders of her own blue city in a blue state.

In 2013, more than two decades after she became a clinic escort, Ulisano was volunteering with the organization she helped found, the Illinois Choice Action Team (ICAT), when she had a thought: What about other groups that need clinic escort vests but can't afford them? She remembered how difficult it had been for ICAT to raise the money to design and print their own vests, and that was in a liberal city. How much harder would it be for volunteers in hostile states?

"I decided to buy vests for any group that wanted them," she explained. "It was just my project . . . The next thing you know, I sent them to [Richmond,] Virginia; Duluth, Minnesota; the Pinkhouse [in Jackson, Mississippi]; orange vests to Louisville[, Kentucky], and the rest took off from there."[53] Ulisano had stumbled on a very real need for clinic escort teams: accessible, quality vests.

That solo project, born out of a tiny seed of an idea, ultimately gave birth to the Clinic Vest Project, a nonprofit organization that provides free vests and training materials to new and longstanding clinic escort teams. When the fledgling team I joined in Englewood, New Jersey, began in late 2013, we used both vests and training materials from the Clinic Vest Project. As of 2021, the organization has donated vests to more than one hundred clinics in forty-two states, Canada, and the United Kingdom.[54]

It may seem small, a box of neon reflective vests. But for Ulisano, it reflects the critical role that her home state now plays as an oasis for this basic care, and the responsibility she feels to this movement.

"I've done a lot of things in this movement, and when I put

the vest on for the first time, my life was profoundly changed in a way that I can't even describe. I knew right then that if I did anything else in this movement, it would be [volunteering as a] clinic escort. And that also was the catalyst behind the Clinic Vest Project. Because when I put it on, I thought, *This is my armor.* It's only made of polyester, and it's not bulletproof, but it's hate-proof and it's judgment-proof."[55]

• • •

My phone buzzed me awake on August 20, 2019. I glanced at it and saw a text from Ashley Gray, the cofounder of my clinic escort team at Metropolitan Medical Associates. "WE THINK WE GOT THE BUFFER ZONE BACK! 3rd circuit reversed the decision!"[56]

I stared at my screen, still waking up. Had I read that right? We hadn't had an active buffer zone at MMA in two years; we had more or less accepted that it was gone, that we were solely responsible for maintaining some semblance of control at the front door of the clinic.

Sure enough, Gray was right. The Third Circuit Court of Appeals overturned the previous ruling, which meant that our buffer zone was still constitutional and therefore still in effect.[57] Protesters would now once again be required to stay at least eight feet away from the clinic's entrance. It wasn't much, but it was a bit of breathing room for patients, and it meant that now we could focus on providing support, rather than just standing guard at the front door.

It felt like a new day. Gray felt it, too. It was time for her and "Jane Roe" to pass the baton. Six years after their first tenuous foray onto the sidewalk, the clinic escort team they had created had grown from three to more than a hundred. In the early days of 2014, the same handful of us were there every single weekend—there just weren't enough of us to spread it out. Now, there were enough that individual escorts could take weeks or even months off, if needed. It was time for some fresh blood, Gray thought. It was time for new leadership to see this amazing volunteer cohort into the next decade.

Gray and "Roe" chose two longtime clinic escorts, both of whom lived in New Jersey and had proven their commitment to the team and the cause. When Andrea Long and Christine Taylor agreed to take over the team in late 2019, they didn't know that they would soon be facing a year unlike any other, as the coronavirus pandemic upended so many customs and established norms in American life. They just knew that the need was still there, that this liberal town in this liberal state, just a stone's throw from New York City, was filled with vicious invective every Saturday morning. And they knew our clinic isn't unique.

"This happens everywhere," Taylor said. "This is not some random, a couple of crazy people at one clinic. This shit happens everywhere in every state and it will continue to happen until people decide that they're going to reclaim their communities."[58]

By the fall of 2020, they were once again outside MMA, enforcing the buffer zone, trying to maintain order, hoping to motivate the community to demand an end to the ongoing harassment at the hands of antiabortion protesters. There was just one small difference: in addition to their matching vests, they all wore masks, gloves, and protective face shields.

Chapter Seven

A Clinic Escort Without a Country

ANN HORN SPENT DECADES OF HER LIFE AT FORT WAYNE Women's Health Organization (FWWHO) in Fort Wayne, Indiana. This clinic had been the sight of turmoil and tragedy, of resistance and resilience, since 1978. Thinking back on the years she spent on the front lines, first as a clinic escort and later as the clinic's sole security guard, she was resolute: "If I could help somebody feel safe, I wanted to do that."[1]

In her decades at FWWHO, she saw Joseph Scheidler, bullhorn in hand, screaming mere feet from her face. She heard cries of "Kill the butcher" ring in her ears.[2] She felt the terror of a bomb threat radiate through her fingers.

Those were the years when the clinic staff and escorts had no one but each other to keep the doors open, when they felt terrified and determined, like they could take on the world because they had to. Horn and her fellow escorts weathered bomb threats. They overcame blockades. They endured bullets flying at providers around the country. They survived it all.

But that was then. Now was a different political climate entirely. In 2011, Indiana passed one of the first TRAP laws in the country, requiring abortion providers to either have admitting privileges at a local hospital or have a "backup" provider who could be named publicly.[3] For the next two years, FWWHO hobbled along, struggling to fulfill the onerous requirement and a series of seemingly endless requests from the Indiana Board of Health.

"[Abortion opponents] had been dragging us through the mud," Horn explained. "They had friends with the state board of health and they were doctoring the records. We could provide [what they asked for], they didn't care. The state would come in and inspect and say, 'Where's your boxes of gloves?' [and] the director would point to them, and they'd write us up anyway."[4]

By December 2013, after losing their backup provider, the clinic had no other option but to cease providing abortions.[5] "All this stuff that they lied about and they drug us through the mud," Horn said. "We just couldn't fight it anymore."[6]

For the first time since 1978, Fort Wayne was without an abortion clinic.

By May 2020, it had been more than six years since Horn had been at FWWHO. In that time, a third of all Indiana abortion clinics had closed their doors.[7] After her clinic closed, Horn tried to stay active, even though there wasn't a clinic near her to support. She went to some pro-choice rallies after Donald Trump's election, but was overcome by a twisted sense of déjà vu. "Oh my god, here we go again," she thought. "Same signs. Same chants. I can't believe we're back where we started."[8]

In a matter of half a decade, Horn went from defending one of the oldest abortion clinics in the Midwest to bemoaning the state of reproductive rights on a national scale. She's no longer a clinic escort or a security guard. Instead, she's home, insulating herself from the coronavirus pandemic, grappling with the legacy of her decades of activism.

Was it enough? What went wrong? How did we get here? How have all of these clinics closed? How did *Roe v. Wade* end up overturned? And if she wasn't defending FWWHO anymore, who was she?

"I fought hard," she muttered to me on the phone. "I did all I could."[9]

• • •

Before *Roe v. Wade* was decided in January 1973, there were really only a handful of places in the country where physicians could provide legal abortion care. Some hospitals and family practice doctors in the few states where it was legalized provided them, but in the 1970s, younger feminists, like Merle Hoffman, put their energy into creating safe, high-quality spaces dedicated to providing abortion care.[10] Choices, her clinic in Queens, New York, was one of them, and it served as a model for how to bring safe abortion care to the masses—through separate clinics.

Abortion rights and women's health advocates successfully fought for legalized abortion, and abortion clinics were heralded as the fruit of that labor. What they failed to foresee was that the existing opposition would not only galvanize around this issue, but refuse to stop finding ways to, if not overturn *Roe v. Wade*, then make it impossible in practice.

Clinic escorts were born out of that backlash. When abortion opponents like Joseph Scheidler targeted abortion clinics and harassed patients, they were doing it to render abortion inaccessible. A central reason that clinics remained open and available for patients was the presence of volunteers like Ann Horn. Now the clinic to which she dedicated decades of her life is gone, and with it legal abortion in northeast Indiana. It is unlikely that it will ever come back.

More than one-third of abortion clinics were forced to close their doors in the past decade, and while not all of them had clinic escort teams, many did.[11] Those former volunteers are, like Horn, without a clinic to serve.

The question that haunted Ann Horn haunts many of these clinic-less escorts, too. The clinic where I volunteered isn't in danger of closing, but that doesn't negate the question: What is a clinic escort without a clinic? If there's no clinic to defend, what can a clinic escort even do?

• • •

On Wednesday, June 27, 2018, the Supreme Court of the United States wrapped up another term. It hadn't been a particularly good one for progressives—the Court upheld Trump's 2017 travel ban on Muslim immigrants, for example.[12] But at least the term was over, and the damage was done for the time being, until Justice Anthony Kennedy dropped a bomb.

That day, he announced that he would step down from the Supreme Court that summer.[13] While Justice Kennedy was appointed by Republican president Ronald Reagan, he had come to serve as the decisive 5–4 swing vote on the Supreme Court, striking down the Texas TRAP law in 2016 and, most famously, writing for the majority in 2015's *Obergefell v. Hodges*, the landmark ruling that legalized same-sex marriage nationwide.[14] Now, Kennedy was handing over his swing vote to President Donald Trump, a man who previously said that there should be "some form of punishment" for people who have abortions if the procedure were made illegal.[15] Once Kennedy was replaced by Brett Kavanaugh, who was accused of sexual assault by several women, including Christine Blasey Ford,[16] many court watchers and abortion rights supporters saw it as the beginning of the end of *Roe v. Wade*.[17] When the Supreme Court decided to take up *June Medical Services v. Russo* for its spring 2020 term, it reinforced the fear that nationwide legal abortion's days were numbered.

At the center of the case was a 2014 Louisiana TRAP law that required abortion providers to have admitting privileges at a local hospital, the same medically unnecessary and onerous requirement that Indiana passed, and that Texas tried to enact in 2013. Louisiana's law was blocked from going into effect by a federal judge, and in June 2016, when Amy Hagstrom Miller emerged victorious on the steps of the Supreme Court, it seemingly signaled the death knell of Louisiana's nearly identical law.

But that was before Donald Trump was elected, before Republicans stole a Supreme Court seat from President Barack Obama, before Neil Gorsuch and Brett Kavanaugh tipped the balance of the Court in a decidedly conservative fashion. *June Medical Services* offered abortion opponents the chance to test the waters of this new Court, and a do-over for *Whole Woman's Health v. Hellerstedt*, which overturned Texas's law. When nearly four hundred congressional Republicans asked the Supreme Court to overturn *Roe v. Wade* and *Planned Parenthood v. Casey*, a 1992 ruling that reaffirmed the right to an abortion, as part of their ruling in *June Medical Services*, any pretense that this case was about "women's health" was immediately eroded.[18]

I spoke with dozens of clinic escorts and abortion rights leaders between March 3, 2020, the day of oral arguments for *June Medical Services*, and June 29, 2020, the day the decision was released. I asked most of them, particularly those in southern and midwestern states that were particularly hostile to abortion rights, how they were feeling, and what they thought might happen. Nearly every single one thought what I thought at the time—that the Louisiana TRAP law would be allowed to go into effect.

Ultimately, Chief Justice John Roberts would prove us wrong. He sided with the Court's liberal justices to strike down the Louisiana law. But it was far from an expansive victory. In his opinion, Roberts made clear that he was striking down the law simply because it was identical to a Texas law struck down by the very same Court just four years prior, a case he felt was "wrongly decided." His opinion did nothing to reaffirm the right to a legal abortion—in fact, it left the door open to future restrictions: "state and federal legislatures [have] wide discretion to pass legislation in areas where there is medical and scientific uncertainty."[19]

At her home in Little Rock, Arkansas, clinic escort Ali Taylor reacted to the decision with a simultaneous wave of relief and twinge of fear.[20] For now, disaster had been averted. Admitting privileges, an insidious abortion restriction, were still unconstitutional, and therefore clinics, including her own Little Rock Family Planning, could stay open. But she knew that antiabortion legislators weren't going to stop at that. They could simply create a new kind of restriction, one that hadn't been tested at the Supreme Court, and use the opening that Chief Justice Roberts provided in his *June Medical Services* ruling to keep it from being blocked.

Mere weeks after that decision, the Eighth Circuit Court of Appeals used Roberts's own arguments to uphold, rather than strike down, four Arkansas abortion restrictions from 2017 that hadn't been allowed to go into effect. They included a ban on the most common procedure for second trimester abortion, severe restrictions on medication abortion, and two invasive requirements of abortion patients, including a mandate that any abortion patient under the age of eighteen have their fetal tissue shared with law enforcement.[21]

It was a devastating blow, revealing a new frontier in the legal fight to protect abortion.

"The good news is, the laws are rejected again, so they're not in effect," Taylor said a few months after the fact. "The laws are being challenged again and again and, at this moment, are not impacting Arkansans."[22]

While that legal fight plays out, Taylor and the rest of the Little Rock Family Planning clinic escorts are continuing on in their pursuit of support for patients. How long they may be able to do that isn't entirely in their control. In March 2021, Arkansas governor Asa Hutchinson signed a six-week abortion ban, the same legislation that swept Alabama, Georgia, Kentucky, and other states in 2016, into law.[23] For now, that's where Arkansas clinic escorts and many in restrictive states will have to stay: stuck in that stressful middle ground, caught between what the law is and where the law might go, hoping for the best while preparing for the worst.

• • •

For nearly thirty years, Justice Ruth Bader Ginsburg, the "Lioness" of the Supreme Court, consistently supported both the need for and the right to abortion care. She was a longtime leader in reproductive rights law. Heralded as "Notorious RBG," she was a frequent dissenting voice in the face of conservative rulings that eroded the rights of the marginalized, like gutting the Voting Rights Act.[24] The news of her passing on September 18, 2020, was salt in an already gaping wound for abortion rights supporters.

When a family member yelped from the next room and said, "Oh god, RBG died," I tried to shake it off as a joke.

"That's not funny," I said.

"I'm not joking."

I stood, frozen with emotional paralysis. It was hard enough to lose Justice Ginsburg and her incredible judicial leadership. But I also

knew that her death now left a vacancy on the already right-tilting
Supreme Court, less than two months before a presidential election.

In her last few days, Justice Ginsburg knew this, too, which was
why she made her request crystal clear: "My most fervent wish is that
I will not be replaced until a new president is installed."[25]

That isn't what happened, of course. Within days of Ginsburg's
death, before she was even buried, President Trump nominated Amy
Coney Barrett to succeed her on the Supreme Court. It was a dia-
bolically absurd nomination, swapping a woman who is publicly and
devoutly anti-choice for *the* judicial heroine of abortion rights. With
just one week to go until the 2020 presidential election, Republicans unilaterally approved her nomination. The Supreme Court
now has a 6–3 conservative bent. Barrett was the perfect Republican
foil for those fearful of *Roe v. Wade*'s future. She's a woman! She's a
working mom! Her meager three years of prior judicial experience
didn't matter—Republicans found what they've been waiting for,
a woman who will overturn *Roe v. Wade* and end nationwide legal
abortion. Even with Joe Biden's victory over Donald Trump in the
2020 presidential election, the Supreme Court will remain a serious
and persistent obstacle to abortion rights for years to come.

It's been a tenuous landscape for abortion clinics for decades, but
now, facing a firm conservative grip on the Supreme Court, clinic
escorts are entering new and uncharted territory. Ann Horn lost her
clinic after years of fighting hostile state regulators, and she won't be
the last. Whether or not *Roe* actually falls, it is undeniable that this
Supreme Court is the most hostile to abortion since its legalization,
and it will undoubtedly uphold severe, draconian restrictions that
will force clinics to close and make it exponentially harder for many
to access abortion.

The wave of grief that I and many other clinic escorts felt in the

wake of Justice Ginsburg's passing was fleeting; we didn't really have
the time to sit and process what this meant, how it felt, how painful
this all was. Clinic escorting emerged as a response to an imperfect
system of plentiful abortion clinics with little legal protection. Now,
that role will have to shift. The problem of ensuring abortion access
with dwindling clinics and increasing restrictions isn't one that clinic
escorts can solve in isolation. Clinic escorts can't just be clinic escorts
anymore—they are integrating with other patchwork approaches to
solving the escalating crisis of abortion inaccessibility.

How Did I Even Get Here?

From the very beginning of her pregnancy in July 2015, Valerie
Peterson had to see a specialist. At thirty-six, Peterson was of "ad-
vanced maternal age" and suffered from high blood pressure, both
of which made her pregnancy high risk. As she neared the end of
her first trimester, she was hopeful. She had been consistently ill
throughout the pregnancy, but the biweekly ultrasounds and specialized genetic testing for the fetus helped put her mind at ease. But at
her sixteen-week ultrasound, she knew something was wrong. After
more than two hours had passed and multiple techs had observed
her, her doctor came in and sat down next to her.

"[He] went through every slide of the ultrasound. When he got
to pictures of my son's brain and showed me what it should have
looked like at that point, as opposed to what it did look like, there
was a significant difference."

The diagnosis was alobar holoprosencephaly, a rare condition in
which the fetus's brain does not split into two halves. "That was the
condition of my baby, and it was one hundred percent incompatible
with life."[26]

The doctor gave her two options: try to carry the pregnancy

to term—resulting in either miscarriage, stillbirth, or a few painful moments of life—or terminate the pregnancy.

Peterson was devastated to learn that her pregnancy wasn't viable. She knew that the pain and trauma of carrying a nonviable pregnancy to term wasn't something she wanted, and she didn't want her son to suffer. She decided to have an abortion.

"Can you admit me to the hospital and take care of the medical procedure?" she asked her doctor. She was already mentally preparing for an imminent trip to the ER, knowing she would come back without a baby.

But Peterson, who had just recently relocated from Kansas to Texas, didn't know about House Bill 2, the 2013 antiabortion legislation that imposed myriad onerous restrictions on abortion, including forcing abortion providers to have admitting privileges at a local hospital and a ban on abortions at twenty weeks.[27] Her doctor explained to her that she couldn't just go to the hospital for an abortion, that she would have to be referred by an abortion provider who had admitting privileges. Instead, she'd have to find her way to one of a handful of remaining operating clinics in a few Texas cities, and because of the backlog, she would likely have to wait for at least three weeks for an appointment. At that point, her pregnancy would likely be past twenty weeks, meaning it would be illegal for her to have an abortion at all.

She broke down.

"I called my aunt who was a trauma nurse and said, 'I can't do this. I don't understand why this is happening.'"

That's when a friend connected Peterson with a clinic in Florida that specialized in providing abortion care for people with later complications in pregnancy. When Peterson called and spoke to the staff, a wave of relief washed over her. Unlike Texas, Florida didn't have a mandatory twenty-four-hour waiting period, nor did it ban

abortions at twenty weeks. She could go to the clinic, have the procedure, and leave, all in the same day. Plus, in addition to the team
of regular clinic escorts outside, the clinic provided individualized
escorts for each patient, people who supported them through the
entire process.

She immediately booked a flight, a hotel room, and a rental car.
In the end, it would cost Peterson $5,000 out of pocket to be able to
have an abortion.[28] She could pay, thankfully. But she knew that so
many others in the same situation wouldn't have that ability. What
would happen to them, she wondered. What would they do?

Since 1976, the federal government has annually renewed the
Hyde Amendment, which bars federal Medicaid funding for abortion care, leaving millions of people stuck to pay the entire cost of
an abortion on their own. As a response, groups of volunteers began
to form collectives to provide financial assistance for abortion patients in need. They called themselves "abortion funds," and they,
like clinic escorts, served as a lifeline, helping to make *Roe*'s promise
more accessible. By 1993, the twenty-two separate abortion funds
across fourteen different states decided to come together. The National Network of Abortion Funds was born.

Today, there are more than seventy abortion funds in their national network. As many states have further restricted abortion by
means of mandatory waiting periods, TRAP laws, and blocking
even private insurance coverage of abortion, the role of abortion
funds has become even more important. What should be covered by
insurance and easily accessible is now a maze of affording transportation, housing, and other logistical challenges. Without abortion
funds, patients without Valerie Peterson's financial safety net would
be out of luck.

Like volunteering as a clinic escort, abortion funds are yet another Band-Aid applied to the gaping wound that years of legislative

and judicial erosion have left in abortion access. They're both about facilitating access where it's difficult, and it's not surprising that there's significant crossover between the two activities. Particularly in states like Texas, which have restricted abortion to the point of inaccessibility, volunteering as a clinic escort and providing abortion funds have both taken on outsize importance and impact.

Steve Leary has a foot in both of those worlds. It's been more than a decade since he lost his wife, Gretchen Dyer, to complications from congenital heart disease. Dyer was a successful screenwriter and playwright, renowned for films like *The Playroom* and *Late Bloomers*.[29] She also taught in the women's studies department at the University of North Texas. In 2005, she, along with some of her students, became a new kind of creator—they founded the Texas Equal Access Fund, or TEA Fund, to fund abortions in the state.[30]

"I never even heard of an abortion fund," Leary said. "When she told me that's what she wanted to do and I'm like, 'People do that?!' She was really smart, kind of visionary . . . she knew this was something that was needed, and she decided she was going to put her time and energy into making it happen."[31]

When she created the TEA Fund in 2005, Dyer could already see the gaps in access for low-income Texans, particularly immigrant women and women of color. This was well before House Bill 2, before TRAP laws emerged, and five years before the beginning of the worst decade for abortion rights since legalization. The TEA Fund provided financial assistance to abortion patients in Texas, but it also integrated another component—clinic escorts.

"I did it with her to support her," Leary recalled. "I've always felt strongly about this issue. I don't really have a personal story of my own, but I've always felt like it was wrong to judge other people and to decide for women what's best for them, their families, and their bodies."

After Dyer passed away in 2009, the TEA Fund stopped facilitating clinic escorts, and Leary retreated from public advocacy. Dyer didn't live to see the fight over House Bill 2, in which Texas state senator Wendy Davis stood in front of her colleagues and filibustered the legislation for thirteen hours. Leary cheered her on, though, feeling his late wife's spirit bounding through Senator Davis's infamous bright pink sneakers. After the legislation took effect, he watched as clinics closed their doors and more Texans attempted to induce their own abortions. Requests for help from the TEA Fund, one of a handful of abortion funds in Texas, increased in the years after House Bill 2.

Alyssa Roscoe (last name changed for privacy) was one of them. When she needed an abortion in 2016, she knew she couldn't afford one. She contacted the TEA Fund, and they agreed to pay for a portion of her procedure at the Whole Woman's Health clinic in Fort Worth. She made multiple appointments—in Texas, you have to wait twenty-four hours between your initial visit and the abortion— during the week. The day of her first appointment, Roscoe tentatively edged her car toward the clinic. She was already on edge as she approached the fence; what if the TEA Fund's payment didn't come through? What if there was a problem with the payment? She had never had an abortion before. Would it hurt? What would it be like?

Then she saw the protesters.

"Whenever I went [to the clinic], there were no escorts, and you would have to park and walk to the clinic by yourself," Roscoe said. "[The protesters] would be yelling at you."[32]

She walked by signs that said WE WANT TO ADOPT YOUR BABY! and BABIES ARE MURDERED HERE! With every step, with every taunt, with every face she saw, she felt certain that no one else should have to endure this to get an abortion, and she wanted to do something.

"That experience of kind of going through it alone, and then my entire process of getting an abortion, I didn't really have any support network at the time . . . Going through that experience, feeling very alienated and shameful, and realizing that's not the way I should have felt through that entire process."[33]

A year after she was a patient there, Roscoe became a clinic escort at Whole Woman's Health. The TEA Fund resumed clinic escort practices in 2017, and Roscoe went from TEA Fund beneficiary to TEA Fund ambassador. The climate outside the clinic remained unchanged; two dozen protesters gathered every day, some wearing MAGA hats, some holding gruesome signs. But she kept showing up.

"Being able to be there, and then we're wearing cute rainbow vests and we're smiling—just meant to be a friendly, comforting presence to them. That was definitely something I felt was really important."[34]

The clinic escorts were severely outnumbered. Some days, it was just her and two other volunteers, trying to support patients past thirty protesters. One of her fellow escorts was Steve Leary.

After the TEA Fund resumed clinic escorting and Donald Trump became the forty-fifth president of the United States, Leary felt called once again to take up the mantle that his wife had created more than a decade earlier. Every time he puts on one of their bright rainbow vests or greets a patient with a warm smile, he once again thinks of his beloved Gretchen Dyer and how she lived her life. People like Roscoe, who relied on the TEA Fund in a moment of need only to give back so much more, are exactly why Dyer created this organization. Putting on that vest means honoring Dyer's legacy, refusing to back down in the face of the unknown.

"She had a heart and lung condition that she was born with, and the doctors told her she wouldn't live very long," Leary remembered. "She knew that she had less time to do what she wanted to do, so she was going to go about doing it. She was fearless."[35]

From the Underground to the Foreground

Despite abortion's illegal status, a vast network of underground activity to ensure access safe to abortion care existed before 1973. Feminist activists, women's health advocates, and health-care providers worked together closely—outside of the law, risking criminalization—to provide abortions to pregnant people in need.

When Carol Downer and her Los Angeles compatriots, as well as the Chicago-based Jane Collective, began facilitating abortions in the late 1960s, they knew that they were breaking the law. That was the point—the law was unjust, and as a result, people were dying from unsafe abortions. As their networks grew and evolved, they closely vetted physicians to ensure that the abortion providers to whom they referred patients were safe and reputable, even if illegal. They also helped garner funds for patients and, once abortion became legal in New York, helped pay for some patients to travel there for a legal abortion. While Downer's cohort stuck to referrals, some members of "Jane" in Chicago learned to provide abortions themselves, creating their own extra-legal network of underground abortion care.

After abortion became legal nationwide, Carol Downer moved from facilitating safe, illegal abortions to operating a legal abortion clinic, and the Jane Collective disbanded—there was no longer a need for underground abortion care. Abortion was now legal nationwide. As abortion clinics proliferated across the nation, it seemed *Roe* had solved the problem for which "Jane" was created.

As of spring 2022, abortion remains technically legal in every single state in the United States, though up to varying points in pregnancy. There's currently no need for a covert, underground operation like the Jane Collective to make safe but illegal abortion accessible. That may change.

The Jane Collective didn't just find (and sometimes even pay for) an abortion; they supported patients in other ways. Some abortion funds, initially created solely to pay for the cost of an abortion, have in recent years begun paying for other costs, like childcare, travel, or hotels, for example. Clinic escorts, typically involved in a short exchange with a patient, have seen in recent years how it isn't just protesters, but also restrictions that hinder access. Walking a patient from their car to the clinic door may not be sufficient anymore. Instead, a new collective has emerged, and like "Jane," it's facilitating access where it otherwise wouldn't exist.

• • •

Steph Black's eyes were glued to her phone. She was desperate to find childcare; not just for an afternoon, she needed someone to stay with a nine-year-old boy for three days. It wasn't for her. It was for a woman who had traveled from Chicago to Washington, D.C., to have an abortion. There was no one in Chicago who could take care of her son, and her health depended on having this abortion. She had to bring him with her.

"Yes!" Black exclaimed as she checked her text messages. "Okay, my friend will watch him for two days. We'll figure out day three later."[36]

Black didn't know this woman or her son. She wasn't a friend or a coworker. She was a total stranger to Black until that very day.

Finally done with her undergraduate education and with more time to devote to the causes that mattered most to her, Black became a clinic escort at Falls Church Healthcare Center in Falls Church, Virginia, in September 2019. She was surprised at how little she actually interacted with patients. "It's like a 'hello/hi' and you just open the door for them," she said. It still felt important to her, even to just be a welcoming face and a supportive figure to patients. She grew accustomed to the limited interaction, imbuing warmth and empathy into every "Hello" and "Welcome" as she opened the door to the clinic.

Three months later, Black heard about a new opportunity—not a replacement for clinic escorting, but an addendum, of sorts. Clinic escorts were responsible for supporting patients *at* the clinic. But what if they couldn't get to the clinic in the first place? What about states that have restricted abortion so severely that patients have to travel hundreds of miles out of state to get to a clinic? These people needed assistance far beyond simply walking past protesters—they needed a structure of support.

When Valerie Peterson needed to travel from Texas to Florida to terminate a nonviable pregnancy, she, unlike many others, had the financial means to do so. But being able to afford it didn't erad-icate the stress and emotional turmoil she experienced. Most people don't understand the ins and outs of getting an abortion until they or someone they love has to face it. For Peterson, having a dedicated clinic escort, assigned to her and her alone, felt like having a life raft. He helped her navigate the process from start to finish, dotting the i's and crossing the t's of aspects of the process that she didn't even know existed. That level of customized, individualized support isn't always possible for abortion patients. But when they are forced to travel great distances, it almost becomes a necessity.

That's why the DMV Abortion Practical Support Network was created. Unlike traditional clinic escorting and defense groups that only support the patient at the clinic, this network does everything else that a patient could possibly need in order to get an abortion. That can include transportation, housing, financial assistance, child-care, and designated personal clinic escorts for patients seeking abor-tion care across the D.C./Maryland/Virginia area.[37]

When Black heard about it, she immediately wanted in. She

signed up to become a part of the all-volunteer collective in December 2019. A few weeks later, she had her first patient: the woman from Chicago, who was facing a severe fetal abnormality and needed a second trimester abortion.

"She was such a sweet woman," Black recalled. "Her family in Chicago wouldn't watch her nine-year-old son," so she had to bring him with her.[38]

Having secured childcare for the woman's son, Black's attention now turned to housing. The collective reserved a hotel for the woman and her son to share for three nights, one that was near the clinic but, because she was undergoing an intensive procedure, would require a driver to and from the clinic each day. Once again, that was Black.

Black had months of experience as a clinic escort, but this was an entirely new dynamic for her. "I clammed up. I was surprised by how uncomfortable I was."[39] She didn't feel judgmental or unsupportive at all; she just had never had such an extensive interaction with a patient. What should she say? What should she *not* say? Should she ask how the woman was feeling? What if the patient didn't want to talk about it? How could she make sure that she was making this woman's experience better, not harder?

Black spent the next three days immersed in this woman's care. She helped the family check into their hotel. She dropped off the woman's son at her friend's house for childcare, then drove the woman to the clinic. She helped the woman out of the car and walked with her, accompanied by the clinic's regular escorts, to the front door. She went back to her car and pulled around to the back of the clinic, spending the next few hours reading a book, waiting for the woman to come back out. She got a text on her phone: "All done coming out in five." She pulled around front, parked, and went into the clinic. She and the patient walked arm-in-arm back to her car, the clinic's main escorts flanking them. She then drove the woman to pick up her son and took them back to the hotel.

Black did this for three days, back-to-back-to-back. The woman opened up to her, sharing how difficult this had all been, how alone she felt, how scared she was to talk to her son about why they were there. Black wasn't just her driver, and she wasn't just her clinic escort—she was a companion. She was a supporter. She was a lifeline.

After the three days, the woman and her son hit the road for their eleven-hour drive back home to Chicago. Black went straight to bed, emotionally and physically exhausted. It had been so hard, and so much work, just to get this woman the abortion she needed to move on with her life and be there for her son, but they had done it. Curled up in bed, Black thought about what it would have been like for this patient if she hadn't been there, and if this network didn't exist. But she was. It did. She drifted off to sleep.

Two weeks later, she got an email. Another patient was coming into town and needed someone to pick them up at the airport. Black took a selfie with her phone, then drafted a text message to the new patient. "Hi, I'm Steph, and I'll be your driver," it read. She included a saved picture of her car, in case the patient had trouble identifying it when she pulled up. As the message whizzed through the ether, Black opened her car door, ready to help another stranger.

• • •

Odile Schalit is no stranger to abortion care—she was a social worker at an abortion clinic in New York City for years. It was there that Schalit saw the human side of abortion, providing direct support services to those who, even in a blue state like New York, had to overcome serious logistical obstacles just to get in the door. She saw the power of collaboration between staff, clinic escorts, abortion funders, and patients to help make access a reality. She saw that accessing an abortion is a collective effort, particularly when it comes to situations like later abortions.

Later-abortion care is uniquely difficult and profoundly misunderstood. According to *Roe v. Wade*, states can restrict abortion after the point of fetal viability, generally what's considered the third trimester of a pregnancy, and forty-three states do.[40] Later abortions, commonly mislabeled "late-term abortions" by abortion opponents, are incredibly rare. Only 1.3 percent of all abortions in the United States occur after twenty-one weeks (the vast majority occur early in pregnancy—according to the Guttmacher Institute, 88 percent of abortions happen within the first trimester. In fact, two-thirds occur at or before eight weeks).[41]

Why would someone need to have an abortion after twenty-one weeks? Why haven't they already figured out they're pregnant and had an abortion? Are they just not paying attention?

Far from it.

Erika Christensen and her husband were delighted when they realized they were pregnant again in 2015, not long after having a miscarriage. The first trimester breezed by without any problems. "Then we started to get some concerning blood test results and my pregnancy was elevated to be high risk," she wrote in *People*. Over the next twelve weeks, complications racked up. Christensen was at thirty weeks when their doctor told them that their fetus wasn't able to swallow, which meant as a baby, he wouldn't be able to breathe. If a baby can't breathe, he can't live.

"We asked our doctor what would happen if I carried to term, and he said I would likely give birth to a baby who would choke for a few moments and then die. We got that information at thirty weeks."[42]

They decided that their least terrible option out of all of their terrible options was to have an abortion. But at that point in her pregnancy, Christensen couldn't just go to the nearest clinic in Manhattan. Instead, they would have to see Dr. Warren Hern, one of the few remaining later-abortion providers in the country. He practices in Boulder, Colorado.

Christensen and her husband would ultimately have to pay $10,000 to have the abortion that neither of them ever wanted to have.[43]

Over time, stories like Christensen's became common for Schalit, but transitioning to facilitating travel for later-abortion care proved a steep learning curve. Providing social work support in an abortion clinic is a targeted, one-on-one endeavor—responding to the needs of a singular patient in that present moment. Now, she had a new venture: the first executive director of the Brigid Alliance, a unique organization that arranges and funds travel for later-abortion care patients. Schalit realized that patients like Christensen aren't just dealing with feelings of trauma and grief; they also have to figure out how to *get* a later abortion. That can feel difficult for anyone under more common circumstances, but for a situation like that of Christensen and others who have later abortions, it can feel downright impossible.

Knowing she couldn't do it alone, Schalit dove into the community: she talked to abortion funds, existing logistical and practical support organizations for abortion like Fund Texas Choice, clinic escorts, and staff members at the few remaining clinics that provide later-abortion care in Maryland, New Mexico, and Colorado.

"[They told] me what worked and what didn't work, and what they felt was needed and what was not needed," she said. "We could talk about redundancy and where redundancy is great and where it's problematic. The success of Brigid has been because we were able to open the door with those relationships and with the heart of collaboration."[44]

When a patient from California needed help traveling to New Mexico for a later abortion due to a severe fetal abnormality, Brigid Alliance, led by Schalit, worked closely with a California-based abortion fund, Access Women's Health Justice, that paid for the cost of the patient's abortion and other practical support, like a personal escort. Brigid paid for the cost of travel and made the hotel and airline reservations. Both organizations filled a specific need and, rather than overlapping with each other, connected to form the basis of the safety net for abortion access that should be created by the law. It shouldn't require a village just to have an abortion. For now, that safety net is created by people like Schalit of Brigid and Tessa Benson of Access Reproductive Justice,[45] and by the dozens of volunteers, escorts, and supporters that work—unpaid—to make up the ground that is lost to current laws' inadequacy, and to sustain that net against whatever hostile legislative and judicial winds are to come.

Since its founding in August 2018, the Brigid Alliance has helped facilitate travel for approximately 1,300 people seeking later-abortion care, an accomplishment that Schalit credits to the incredible network—of which she is now a part—that crosses boundaries and borders to make abortion access possible. As the ground continues to shift underneath escorts' feet, it's clear that the patchwork system to facilitate abortion access—abortion funds, practical support, and clinic escorts—isn't going away. Instead, it will have to become more adept and more collaborative in order to bridge the growing divide.

"Having been a social worker in a clinic, working day in and day out, [I felt] incredibly powerless, like I couldn't prevent or solve any of the problems that happened before my patient came into my room," Schalit explained. "Now, I get to be a part of this huge network that exists beyond those four walls, that is not only actively participating in trying to help that same patient to get to that social worker and that clinic, and make sure they get there safely, but is participating in the activism and the advocacy that will hopefully one day make it so that person doesn't have to travel at all to get their care and can just go to a town down the street."[46]

The network that Schalit is now a part of will have its hands full in the years to come; it already does, and it's the reason why the United States still has what little abortion access it does. Since the beginning of legal abortion in the United States, there have been systemic barriers to abortion care for too many, particularly low-income women and women of color, whom the Hyde Amendment, which bars federal funding of abortion care, has disproportionately affected.[47] As clinics continue to close and increasingly draconian restrictions are upheld by a conservative Supreme Court, those barriers will only grow more onerous, and the response from both current and former clinic escorts will have to rely on the collaborative network they have developed with abortion funds and practical support groups, if access to safe abortion is to continue.

Renee Bracey Sherman hasn't been a clinic escort in years. But her time as a clinic escort helped inform some of her later advocacy work with the National Network of Abortion Funds and We Testify, the powerful spin-off organization that she leads, which promotes and supports abortion storytellers. Sherman credits volunteering as a clinic escort with helping her shape how she approaches her work as executive director of We Testify, helping to protect and support others who, like her, have had an abortion and want to share their stories.

"For me, it was a good practice in nonengagement work," Sherman said. "Talking to storytellers, especially if they're going to be at a rally and [antiabortion protesters] will be there, [it helps me] talk to them about what nonengagement looks like. [Clinic escorting] prepped me to be a defender for storytellers, to be a security guard. I'm their personal assistant and hyper-vigilant."[48]

Without a legal system to support them or a clinic to call their own, some clinic escorts might find that Sherman's transition will ultimately reflect their own. They may gravitate to a collective like the DMV Abortion Practical Support Network or the Brigid Alliance. The central theme of all of these activities, from volunteering as a clinic escort to funding abortions to booking travel for abortion patients, is community. Having an abortion can be an extremely isolating experience—it's stigmatized, and we don't talk about it; therefore, if you need an abortion, you may not know who to ask or what to do. The Jane Collective took the isolation out of finding a safe, illegal abortion. Once abortion was legalized, abortion clinics proliferated, and with them the assumption that they would meet that need for community and collective support. Ultimately, with the strength and endurance of abortion opponents, clinics became a battleground. The work of community-building around abortion care, of destigmatizing and humanizing people who have abortions, can't be the sole responsibility of embattled clinics and providers. Telling stories, driving patients, paying for gas money, walking someone from their car to the clinic—these may seem small, but they are profoundly meaningful to someone who needs them.

As conservative states continue to restrict and ban abortion—in late April 2021, the country saw a record twenty-eight abortion restrictions signed into law in a single *week*—building and maintaining a community of support for abortion care will become even more essential to help people get basic care. Whether walking someone past a group of protesters or booking someone a hotel room, the essential work is the same—and clinic escorts are already doing it.

Chapter Eight

How Do You Solve a Problem Like Abortion?

IN 1986, AFTER NINE YEARS AS DIRECTOR OF AN ABORTION clinic in Pittsburgh, Pennsylvania, Jeanne Clark was ready for a change. She loved running the clinic—managing the staff, supporting the patients, serving the community. She also experienced the darker side of working in the abortion rights movement. Thankfully, no one was home when her house was firebombed. Another time, someone opened fire on the house—though her son was home, he was mercifully unhurt. But she wasn't fleeing the movement or the work. She was ready to apply her firsthand experience as both a clinic director and a victim of antiabortion terrorism to the broader fight to end antiabortion harassment and violence. When Eleanor Smeal of the National Organization for Women (NOW) offered her a job as press secretary, specifically focusing on abortion rights, she didn't hesitate.[1]

Her timing was prescient, because a more widespread version of the violence she herself had endured was on the horizon. Operation Rescue began within a few months of Clark's joining NOW, and clinic blockades became routine. Her job description transformed—she was now tasked with informing the media of the reality of abortion access in America and the effects of the protesters' hostility and aggression. It wasn't just about defending abortion's legality, but about trying to tell a broader story of what access to legal abortion required and why the barriers to it were unacceptable. That meant focusing on the human side, rather than the political side, of abortion.

> We made the woman visible in the issue. The antiabortion forces' main goal was to have abortions done on invisible women with visible fetuses. We gave visibility to women. We gave that control to women. We gave that visual route and I saw it firsthand, how the majority of people, women and men, became more and more accepting. They might not vote on it. They might not think about it that much. But I watched that happen.[2]

As isolated blockades turned to the Summer of Mercy, the media narrative shifted, and with it the political pendulum. Clark worked tirelessly to support an effort by a Melbourne, Florida, abortion clinic to beat back rampant and chaotic protests, and they won a significant victory at the start of 1994 when the Supreme Court okayed the use of racketeering laws to sue the protesters.[3] A few months later, she cheered the passage of the FACE Act, heralding it as a new moment for abortion access. The law was still on the side of abortion rights.

In late July 1994, mere days after Dr. John Bayard Britton and James Barrett were gunned down outside the Ladies Center in Pensacola, Florida, Clark's phone rang. On the other end was Eleanor Smeal. The New Woman Medical Center in Jackson, Mississippi, was under siege by abortion opponents, and Dr. Joseph Booker Jr., the abortion provider, was receiving threats. As a result, a local group of abortion rights supporters had emerged, calling themselves Pro-Choice Mississippi. They had the will to help, but they needed organizing, training, and resources. Would she come help?

Clark thought about the risks to her safety just long enough to pack a bag, kiss her family, and book a flight.

In Jackson, Clark helped local activists organize a group of clinic escorts and defenders, creating a fortress that protected the clinic on the three days each week that Dr. Booker performed abortions. "I spent my forty-fifth birthday in a bulletproof vest in the Mississippi heat in August," she recalled.

The clinic stayed open and Dr. Booker remained unharmed. Safe, legal abortions continued in Jackson.

After the siege died down, Clark returned to her home in Pittsburgh. Over the next few years, she watched as activists continued to step in to protect abortion access where the law stopped. She witnessed the law strengthening in some cases, with the passage of national FACE Act and local ordinances in Pittsburgh to solidify abortion rights. At one point, she was hopeful that eventually the "war" would be won and legal abortion would be protected.

Today, though, that Jackson clinic that Clark defended is long gone. The FACE Act? Unevenly unenforced. And the racketeering case against antiabortion protesters that Clark helped support? The Supreme Court tossed out that conviction in 2003.[4]

"No victory is really permanent if you take your eye off the ball for a second," she said. The question now is, can we even see the ball if it's moving this fast?

• • •

The sun had long since set on October 26, 2020, by the time Amy Coney Barrett (no relation to Dandy or James Barrett) stood on the

South Lawn of the White House. Dressed in a black dress and pearls, she stood across from Associate Justice Clarence Thomas, one of the longest-serving and most reliably conservative members of the Supreme Court. She placed her left hand on a Bible and her right hand in the air, and repeated the cued words from Justice Thomas. Within a matter of seconds, Barrett became the 115th member of the United States Supreme Court, just eight days before the 2020 presidential election.[5]

Earlier that day, she was confirmed on a strictly partisan vote line by Senate Republicans to replace Justice Ruth Bader Ginsburg,[6] whose judicial philosophy and legal bona fides couldn't be more different. Barrett, a woman with only three years of judicial experience, subscribes to a deeply conservative view of the Constitution. Most alarmingly for abortion rights advocates, she has explicitly called for *Roe v. Wade* to be overturned.[7] A mere week before Donald Trump's fate as a one-term president was sealed, he managed to ensure that his administration's legacy of fanaticism and opposition to legal abortion would long outlast his four traumatic years in office.

The United States had just exited the most disastrous decade for abortion rights since it was legalized in 1973. Even before *Dobbs*, this decade was well on track to be even more catastrophic. After four years of a presidency that nearly ended democracy, aided and abetted by congressional Republicans who did more to investigate a fake Planned Parenthood scam than possible treason by the president himself, it was already obvious that abortion rights have been in crisis for years. But now, they're in a free-fall. When the Supreme Court overturned *Roe v. Wade* in June 2022, it didn't just end the constitutional right to an abortion—it sentenced millions of people, across vast swaths of the South and the Midwest—to institutionalized suffering and dehumanization. As of November 2022, abortion is currently illegal in thirteen states. According to the Guttmacher

Institute, abortion could be banned in as many as 26 states once the dust settles in our post-Roe reality.

The impossible is here. We are living in it. How do we get out of this?

There's no magic potion or silver bullet that will save abortion rights. There never really was. *Roe v. Wade* was a significant step, but while many abortion rights supporters assumed it was the end, it was really just the beginning of a much longer fight. There isn't a simple law that Congress can pass that will make it all go away. The crisis in abortion access is multilayered, integrated with racism, poverty, and deep, abiding misogyny. We have to do the very taxing and messy work of really looking at how we've ended up here, and what we can do differently now. We have to reckon not just with America's laws, but with the limitations of those laws—and how, too often, the law penalizes the marginalized. We have to take a long, hard look at how and why we've allowed this issue, an experience that one in four women in America have had in their lifetimes, to be framed as something worthy of shame and derision. Abortion isn't just legal; it's common. Why don't we treat it that way?

The Limits of the Law

This could be the moment I die, Erin Matson thought as she shuffled through the darkness toward the front door of the townhouse occupied by Germantown Reproductive Health Services in Maryland in the summer of 2011. She and a half dozen other volunteers flanked Dr. LeRoy Carhart, a one-time assistant of Dr. George Tiller and one of the last four later-abortion providers in the United States. Law enforcement had been outside the clinic earlier in the day, fending off approximately fifty antiabortion protesters from Operation Rescue. The police had gone, and now, after sunset, Dr. Carhart needed to get inside the clinic to continue a multiday procedure on a patient. How much could the law protect them now? They were all alone, in the dark, right in the sight line of dozens of the most dedicated and diehard abortion opponents.

"There had already been real concerns about suspicious looking objects, [in addition to] all of the threats [that Dr. Carhart received]," Matson recalled. "No one was there except the antis, and about six to eight of us [clinic escorts]. Dr. Carhart had to walk with these people watching and no one else there . . . from his car into the door of his clinic, and that's probably thirty-five to forty feet."[11]

Then just over thirty years old, Matson was already a seasoned clinic escort and defender, and she knew that the threats against Dr. Carhart weren't necessarily idle. By showing up to support him, she and the other volunteers were putting their health and safety at risk. By the summer of 2011, it had been twenty years since the Summer of Mercy blockades shut down abortion clinics in Wichita, Kansas. Barack Obama was president. The Affordable Care Act, which required health insurance companies to cover contraception without a copay, was beginning to roll out. Two new female justices had already been added to the Supreme Court during Obama's tenure, including the first ever Hispanic and Latina member of the Court, Justice Sonia Sotomayor.

It was also two years after the tragic murder of Dr. George Tiller, a central target of the Summer of Mercy. Only four later-abortion providers were left in the country, spread out across New Mexico, Colorado, and Maryland. All abortion providers were on edge and taking extra precautions. Operation Rescue/Operation Save America decided that the summer of 2011 was once again their moment— they announced a new Summer of Mercy, but not in Wichita. There was no need there anymore after Tiller's murder. This time, they chose Germantown, Maryland, and Dr. Carhart.[12]

Carhart, who in 2011 had just turned seventy, had already weathered years of harassment and violence. His farm burned down in a mysterious fire in 1991, the same year as the original Summer of Mercy, killing seventeen horses, a cat, and a dog. He has been defiant in the face of ongoing harassment and the death of his dear friend Dr. Tiller. "They're at war with us," he told *Newsweek* in 2009. "We have to realize this isn't a difference of opinions. We need to fight back."[13]

He had also seen how the law could be used to help and hurt abortion access. The Obama administration took a more aggressive approach to enforcing the FACE Act than the previous Bush administration, a heartening sign on the federal level.[14] But Carhart had also been chased out of the state of Nebraska, where he had provided abortions for years. After Tiller's murder, he started performing later abortions there as well,[15] until the state legislature responded by passing the first twenty-week abortion ban in the nation in 2010.[16]

Now, his clinic in Maryland was about to experience an onslaught from the same people who rubbed shoulders with Scott Roeder, the man who had assassinated his dear friend Dr. Tiller.[17]

The Summer of Mercy revival brought a fraction of the protesters that the original did, and the clinic worked closely with local and federal law enforcement to ensure security. But on the few occasions when law enforcement wasn't there, Matson and the other volunteers were—they picked up where the law left off.

"We walked around [Dr. Carhart] in a circle, just surrounding him as he walked in [to the clinic]," she said. "I really thought, they might shoot right now. We just don't know."[18]

In the end, no one did shoot. After weeks of abortion opponents trying unsuccessfully to sow chaos, no one got hurt, and no one was ultimately denied care. Matson walked away from that experience with a renewed sense of purpose and defiance, one that wasn't tied to an election or a politician but to a core value. The myopic focus on simply saving *Roe* and winning elections wasn't working.

> [Saving *Roe*] alone does not solve the problem. All the ener-
> gy [from abortion supporters] seemed to be getting poured
> into defeating a guy who says, "Rape rules because then you
> have a baby out of it,"[1] but that's not a vision, and that's not
> expanding access to care . . . Look where we are now.[19]

That perceived lack of passionate, full-throated embrace of abortion led Matson and Pamela Merritt to cofound Reproaction, a direct-action group for abortion rights and reproductive justice. Reproaction isn't interested in quietly lobbying or backdoor poli-cymaking, but in "going on unapologetic offense and ending the defensive crouch on reproductive rights."[20]

If the law won't do it, then activists will.

• • •

I was born in 1985, more than a decade after *Roe v. Wade* was decided. I've never lived in a country with illegal abortion. And yet, for as long as I've been alive, safe and legal abortion has been under attack.

I was just two years old when Randall Terry led the first block-ade of an abortion clinic in Cherry Hill, New Jersey. Dr. John Bayard Britton, the abortion provider who was murdered alongside his clinic escort James Barrett, traveled every week from my home-town of Jacksonville, Florida, to continue providing abortions in

---

1. In 2012, Missouri Senate Republican candidate Todd Akin claimed that abor-tion because of rape wasn't necessary because "If it's a legitimate rape, the female body has ways to try to shut that whole thing down." His comment and the sub-sequent backlash likely contributed to his loss to Claire McCaskill, a Democrat.

Pensacola after Dr. David Gunn's murder. In June 1992, weeks after I completed kindergarten, the Supreme Court upheld the constitutional right to an abortion in *Planned Parenthood v. Casey* but weakened existing precedent that helped pave the way to this crisis point.[21] When the Supreme Court upheld a ban on a common second trimester abortion procedure in *Gonzales v. Carhart* in 2007, I was still in college.[22] Just three years later, as I rang in my twenty-fifth birthday, so too came the start of the most rampant, restrictive anti-abortion decade in modern memory.

I'm in my midthirties now, and this dramatic erosion of abortion rights has happened within my short lifetime.

Now, here we are: we've lost *Roe v. Wade*, a ruling that had the benefit not only of judicial precedent but of public support. Seven in ten Americans support legal abortion, yet it's still a fresh political fight, a never-ending ideological war, a charged issue for supporters and opponents, a rallying cry.[23]

But even with *Roe* in place, abortion access was already in crisis.

If we take a surface-level look at the 1992 *Planned Parenthood v. Casey* decision, the Supreme Court did technically uphold a person's constitutional right to an abortion. But it also allowed states to restrict abortion *before* the point of fetal viability, as long as those restrictions don't place an "undue burden" on the person seeking an abortion.[24] However, the Court failed to define what an "undue burden" is, and in doing so, they opened the door for some restrictions, like parental consent laws, that helped fuel the tidal wave of antiabortion legislation from 2010 through 2019.[25]

Is it an undue burden when hundreds of protesters block the entrance to your health-care appointment? Or if you have to have a stranger shield your face to protect you from being photographed by protesters? Is it an undue burden to be forced to drive hundreds of miles to a clinic on a spare tire, hoping that it lasts? Is the burden undue if you have to decide between eating for a few days or paying for an abortion? What about if you have to terminate a wanted pregnancy because of fetal inviability, but you can't do it in your own state because you're past the pregnancy cutoff?

Clinic escorts have seen, up close, the burdens big and small, legal and personal, that hinder abortion access. The act of volunteering as a clinic escort itself was born out of one of those challenges, of protesters harassing abortion patients and trying to shut down clinics with their bodies.

Since the early days of *Roe*, there have been intentional and continual barriers to that care, burdens that are manufactured to make having an abortion as onerous as possible. Laws like the Hyde Amendment,[26] which bars federal funding of abortion care, work in tandem with protesters from 40 Days for Life, to make abortion *technically* legal, but *practically* inaccessible. Laws like the FACE Act, which made it a federal crime to block access to a clinic, and clinic escorts work together to make walking into an abortion clinic less physically and emotionally fraught for patients.

Laws can do great harm and great good. So can people.

Abortion isn't just a legal issue—it's a practical one. The stated intent of a law doesn't adequately account for its effects. Valerie Peterson had to travel to another state to have an abortion because of the restrictive provisions that Texas enacted in 2013. She wasn't technically banned from having an abortion, but what if she had been someone who couldn't afford to fly to Florida? That's the ultimate effect of that legislation.

Abortion is about more than just bodies on the line—it's someone's future, their dreams, their lives. When abortion is reduced to a mere political fight, we miss that, and we miss the very real stakes when access to it is denied. We also miss the underlying truth that legal abortion has never been freely accessible, not to everyone, and we fail to see the reason it has been able to limp along for as long as it has—because everyday people gave their time, resources, and sometimes their lives to keep it that way.

The law isn't the beginning or the end of abortion access. For decades, clinic escorts have been a neon-vested visualization of the law's limits. As we move into a post-*Roe* America, the black-and-white focus on abortion's legality will only serve to leave the most marginalized behind.

• • •

When Benita Ulisano sees a protester blocking the entrance to FPA in Chicago, her first call likely isn't to the FBI or the Justice Department but to local law enforcement. While state and federal legislators are largely responsible for creating the laws meant to protect abortion access at the clinic door, local police are the primary means of enforcing those laws.

However, most of the clinic escorts with whom I spoke echoed my own experience with calling police on protesters—it rarely helps. Some don't care about the city's given laws to protect abortion clinics, while others just don't seem to know the laws at all. Clinic escorts are there because the law doesn't extend far enough to truly protect this constitutional right, yet clinic escorting is often perceived as one side of a two-sided debate, rather than the service that it is. I was targeted once by a protester who claimed I had harassed him by putting my hand up to block him from filming a patient. When a police officer insisted that I share my home address for the police report, I said I was afraid to give the protesters that kind of information, that I could be harassed or even subject to violence in my own home. His response? "Well, you should have thought of that before you came out here."

Some clinics, like Kromenaker's Red River Women's Clinic in Fargo, North Dakota, say they have a solid working relationship with local law enforcement. They may be the exception, rather than the rule. But there are some states and cities that do provide additional legal protection for clinics, like New York City's buffer zone ordinance or Chicago's bubble zone law, both of which technically require protesters to maintain solid distances from patients. How are those laws enforced? By calling the police.

Suppose Ulisano watches a protester get right in the face of a patient, following her all the way to the door, a clear violation of the city's law requiring protesters to maintain eight feet of space from the patient at all times. Should she call the police? Most likely, she won't. She knows that at most they'll give a word of warning to the protesters and leave.

Relying on the apparatus of the law to protect abortion access isn't likely to bring about the results that Ulisano and that patient want to see.

There's another concern in the back of Ulisano's mind, one that clinic staff have to wrestle with every time something illegal happens: Would calling the police make the clinic feel more or less safe to the patients? For patients of color, particularly Black people and undocumented immigrants, the sight of a police car outside an abortion clinic doesn't necessarily bode safety, but potential for harm, deportation, or even death. The presence of law enforcement outside a clinic could discourage these people, already marginalized and targeted for criminalization, from accessing the care they need.

Sometimes the law is a friend, and sometimes it's a foe.

If providers are meeting patients where they are, sometimes that means accepting that law enforcement is a hindrance rather than a help. In more conservative areas or more restrictive states, the law can pit even potentially friendly police officers against abortion providers. Clinics can serve as a visible focal point for hostility and community tensions around abortion and policing. Clinic escorts sometimes get caught up in this as well. It's hard for patients to always understand what the bright neon vests mean— some patients assume clinic escorts are protesters or even members of law enforcement—and, as I've experienced myself, clinic escorts are sometimes regarded by police as instigators, or at least as part of the problem.

If the law can't or won't protect the clinics, how can we still protect abortion access?

• • •

One answer is to take abortion out of the clinic and hand it directly to the people who need it. During Operation Rescue's heyday, the only way to get an abortion was to physically go to a provider, most likely at an independently owned clinic (even today, the majority of abortions take place at an independent clinic, rather than at a Planned Parenthood[27]). But that's not the case anymore. In fact, up to twelve weeks of pregnancy, a patient likely may not even need to set foot in a clinic or hospital to have a safe abortion. Medication abortion, a combination of two medications, mifepristone and miso- prostol, allows people to safely terminate pregnancies at home.

In some states, like Oregon, that's easily done via telemedicine. An abortion provider prescribes you a medication abortion virtually and continually checks in as you take the series of five pills to safely terminate your pregnancy. However, abortion opponents have re- alized how potentially revolutionary telemedicine abortion is and have moved to curb this safe medical practice. Before *Roe* was even overturned, nineteen states required the physician to be physically present when prescribing medication abortion, which renders tele-medicine abortion impossible.[28]

The internet could be a game-changer for abortion, though. It is now legal in thirteen states to order medication abortion online and receive it by mail.[29] Even in states where the law is unclear, people still seek out medication abortion online. It's one of the many hats that clinic escorts are now wearing—trying to help people access medication abortion online as covertly and safely as possible.

Steph Black, the clinic escort and practical support volunteer who drives patients to their abortion appointments in Washing-ton, D.C., also supports the facilitation of online medication abor-tion. She's one of the lead ambassadors for Plan C, an organization through the National Women's Health Network that works to de-medicalize medication abortion and help prospective patients find abortion pills.[30] Black was trained by medical professionals on the ins and outs of medication abortion and how to provide quality infor-mation to those in need. Black doesn't prescribe medication abortion or purchase it—she just serves to help provide people in need with the information they seek.

"I understand all the protocol of how to manage an abortion," she explained. "I can give information and advice—that is neither medical or legal advice—about self-managed abortion, in safe ways. I think there's a lot of people who are stepping up and starting to prepare for the end of *Roe*."[31]

Plan C is just one of many options for safe, online medication abortion provision. There's also Aid Access, a private initiative of Dr. Rebecca Gomperts, who gained international notoriety for creating Women on Waves, in which she sailed her boat to countries where abortion was illegal or heavily restricted and safely performed them at sea, beyond international borders. Aid Access ships medication abortion to people who cannot access it. Patients who are less than nine weeks pregnant can fill out an online consultation form and receive guidance from their team of doctors about purchasing medication abortion online.[32]

People have been increasingly turning to these online support systems amid the coronavirus pandemic. Within the first few weeks of the pandemic in the United States, Aid Access saw a 27 percent increase in the rate of request for pills.[33] The realities of the pandemic—the need to social distance, the fear of going into indoor facilities—have made medication abortion a more desirable and feasible option.

The benefits of easy, accessible, online medication abortion must also be balanced with the risks. People, particularly women of color, have already been criminalized for self-managing their abortions, or even for having a miscarriage. Overzealous prosecutors have used feticide laws, originally created as a form of extra protection for pregnant people and their fetuses against assault and battery during pregnancy, to criminalize women of color for self-managing their own abortion. In 2013, Purvi Patel, an Indiana woman, was convicted of feticide and child neglect and sentenced to thirty years in prison after she took medication abortion while pregnant.[34] Her conviction was eventually overturned by a judge who railed against using feticide laws to criminalize women for self-managing their abortions.[35] But that hasn't stopped some prosecutors. Four years after Patel's conviction, Latice Fisher, a Black mother of three, was indicted for second-degree murder in Mississippi after she gave birth to a stillborn fetus because she had previously conducted a Google search for medication abortion. The charges against her were dropped a year later.[36]

Even when abortion law seems black and white, it rarely is.

The risks of purchasing medication abortion online aren't going away. But trying to control medication abortion may be like trying to put the genie back in the bottle.

"Nothing scares the antiabortion movement like self-managed abortion with pills does," Erin Matson said. "Because what can they do? What are they going to do? Are they going to bomb everyone's house? Not knowing what's inside someone's medicine cabinet. They can't control it."[37]

If someone really wants an abortion, they will find a way to get one. Abortion, regardless of legality, should be safe. As advocates and lawyers work to defend or even change the law to protect abortion rights in the courts and legislatures, we need look no further than the legacy of clinic escorts to see the pathway forward for abortion: where the law ends, people like Benita Ulisano pick up the chain.

"I have refused to accept 'post-*Roe*' ideas," she said defiantly. "I'm not going there because I truly believe that even though all of this bad stuff is happening, I do think, in the end, we're going to prevail . . . I refuse to believe that abortion will become illegal in this country. I'm not going to accept that and I'm going to fight whatever fight is needed to prevent that."[38]

"I think we're going to win," Erin Matson told me, her voice calm and clear. "I think it's going to be really, really hard, and it's going to get worse before it gets better. But I believe so strongly in the capacity of people to do what is best for themselves."[39]

Amy Hagstrom Miller, the CEO of Whole Woman's Health who won the landmark Supreme Court case against a Texas TRAP law in 2016, refuses to give up hope, either.

I think hope is the biggest rebellion. I believe that humans are creative and innovative and can prevail, that ultimately the majority of people are good. It's helpful to work in a field where, literally, I would say we're in the business of second chances. People get to have these moments in our work that are much beyond the political—how thankful people are, and how real those relationships are, that we really help people get the care that they need and step back into the life they dreamed of. It's pretty rewarding. That's where the hope comes from.[40]

I believe in the capacity of people to do what is best for others, because I've seen it. I've lived it. Whatever the law says and however it is applied, we still have the power to support each other. We still have the power to make safe abortion a tangible and accessible reality for everyone. There's power in the gray.

The Humanity of Abortion

Liz Gustafson first decided to become a clinic escort at the Hartford GYN Center in Hartford, Connecticut, in 2017, soon after Donald Trump was inaugurated. She loved being a part of a community, a consistent, visible display of support for those who needed abortions. Even after she started working for NARAL, the abortion rights advocacy organization, she continued supporting the clinic escorts.

"If something happened, they'd call me if they wanted me to come down to have someone outside to help document everything."[41]

Three months into her new job, she found out she needed an abortion. She could easily just go to the clinic where she volunteered; she already knew and trusted the staff. But the thought of having to walk past the protesters who already knew her name was too much. She just wanted to get in and get out, with as little fanfare as possible, and she didn't want to make the scene outside the clinic any more chaotic than it already was. That's what every patient deserved, and it's what so few of them could access. She might not be able to avoid protesters, but she could at least avoid the protesters who knew her. She opted for another clinic.

"I was so worried about the opposition finding out and using it to hurt the clinic, hurt our efforts, go after our boss [at NARAL], go after my family," she said. "Stigma manifests in so many ways."

Gustafson was sure she wanted to have an abortion, and she didn't regret having one. But she still felt the stinging nettle of stigma about having one. She knew what abortion opponents were capable of, and she knew how easily her name and face could end up posted online. She wasn't ashamed that she had an abortion, but she still felt reticent to be publicly identified as someone who had had one.

Despite nearly half century of legalization and commonality—one in four people who can get pregnant in the United States will have an abortion in their lifetime[42]—abortion remains a socially stigmatized procedure. Gustafson isn't alone in experiencing abortion stigma. Research shows that two out of three people who have abortions anticipate stigma if others become aware of it, and 58 percent feel they need to keep their abortion secret from friends and family.[43] Research also shows that more than 95 percent of people who have abortions don't regret the choice.[44]

What does it say when most people are glad that they had an abortion, but afraid to let anyone know?

"It was just a really bizarre feeling, being in the movement but then within the movement," Gustafson said. "I find only in private conversations do people talk to me about their abortions."[45]

Even those who devote their lives to defending abortion rights are still subject to the pervasive social stigma around this health-care procedure. How can anyone possibly avoid it when people are screaming that abortion is murder and those who have one will burn in hell?

We treat abortion like a shameful secret, something *other* people do, something *I* would never do. Even if you have, even if you know someone who has, even if you may one day need to—we don't talk about abortion as if it's the common, normal experience that it really is.

Think about it. How often do you hear the word "abortion" in everyday conversation? When is the last time you saw a real human-interest news story about a person who had an abortion, and what that was like for them? How often do you hear about abortion outside of political restrictions or bans? What kind of abortion stories do you see in the media you consume?

In 2013, researchers found that, of the 310 American television and film plotlines that contained abortion in the previous *century*, just above half resulted in an abortion, and 13.5 percent ended in the death of the person who sought an abortion.[46] Legal abortion is fourteen times safer than childbirth, and has a mortality rate of less than one per 100,000 procedures.[47]

In recent years, television and movies have begun to tell more honest, complex stories about abortion. In 2019, as conservative states passed abortion bans at an unprecedented rate, Hollywood documented more abortion stories than researchers had ever seen in a single year.[48] Yet for every episode of abortion-positive television, like when Annie has a perfectly quotidian abortion in Hulu's *Shrill*,[49] or when Abbi and Ilana volunteer as clinic escorts in *Broad City* and mock the protesters for their hypocrisy,[50] there's also an episode of *Black Mirror* that confuses emergency contraception with medication abortion, when they are very clearly two different kinds of medicine.[51] In *Obvious Child*, needing an abortion becomes a part of a sweet rom-com, bringing the two leads together in a romantic, post-abortion cuddle on the couch. Juxtapose that with *Juno*, which, while tenderly and comically dealing with adolescent pregnancy, also portrays antiabortion protesters as well-meaning, sweet, docile teenagers and clinic staff as absent-minded, careless hacks. This isn't just inaccurate—it distorts how we see the very real threats that abortion staff and patients face, and it normalizes protesters' opposition to abortion as well-intentioned, rather than hostile.

That stigma helps keep the experience of abortion relegated to the shadows, and it reinforces abortion as being solely a political issue, rather than a fundamentally human one. Socially, abortion is legal but it's rarely acceptable. That allows protesters to continue to harass patients unimpeded, and it keeps otherwise completely devoted advocates like Gustafson from fully embracing what she did when she opted for an abortion: she made what she felt was the right decision for her own life.

Instead, she had to worry about whether protesters would photograph her, harass her, or even attack her. She wondered if they would find her phone number or address, whether they would show up at her home. She didn't know if she'd be able to have an abortion and go on with her life, or if she'd be followed or harassed by abortion opponents everywhere she went. She had to worry about her colleagues' safety at the Hartford GYN Center, and her own.

That shouldn't be a concern for anyone seeking an abortion. No one should have to fear for their safety, and no one should have to fear judgment, either. Yet as long as we continue to avoid talking about abortion in plain and open terms, unapologetically, those tragedies will continue to be a part of patients' decision-making and overall experience.

There's so much we miss about this issue in our aversion to talking openly about it. We miss the nuance and complexity of people's lives, and the possibility for compassion and empathy for those who are sometimes making difficult or complicated decisions about what's best for them and their families. We lose the ability to connect to each other in moments of confusion and uncertainty. Most pointedly, we cede ground to those who want to take away this most basic right when we act as though it's not really worth protecting.

"Everyone loves someone who has had an abortion," Renee Bracey Sherman, activist and former clinic escort, likes to say. "And if you think you don't, they just haven't shared their story with you yet."[52]

If, before you read this book, you didn't know anyone who has had an abortion, you do now. The next time you hear a legislator or pundit talking about *Roe v. Wade* or abortion as a political football, think of Valerie Peterson or Liz Gustafson. Think of women like Paula Schneider, who buried her abortion for decades, until she walked a terrified young woman into a clinic and found herself blurting out the words "I've had an abortion."

That's what this fight is really about.

• • •

One afternoon in May 2019, after I spoke at a rally about abortion rights and my experience as a clinic escort, a woman came up to me, curious to know more. She asked how to get involved and for some resources. She asked how long I'd been volunteering, and how many people I've walked into the clinic in that time. I shrugged and said, "Quite a few, I'm sure." She paused, and met my gaze.

"Do you remember them?"

I stopped and thought about it. I have no idea how many people I've walked into the clinic, and truth be told, I wouldn't recognize 99 percent of them if they walked right up to me. I don't know their names. I don't know their situations. I don't know what they do for a living. I don't know where they live, what their favorite color is, what band they love. I really don't know anything about them. I don't really remember them.

But they do stay with me. When I think about how bleak the landscape is for abortion rights, or when I feel fear or self-doubt in making any kind of life decision, the patients I've served are present, lingering in my hippocampus. Every time I feel burned out or think about giving up on this fight, I remember that putting my body on the line for another person, as painful and difficult as it was on the worst days, has always been worth it.

"Every patient we get in the door is a victory," said Laura Horowitz, a thirty-year clinic escort in Pittsburgh. "Every patient we get in the door is a woman's life, a person's life, that is going to unfold the way that person wants it to, no matter what choice they end up making."[53]

The patients we serve stay with all of us, because that's the spirit of what we do. In those sixty or so seconds before they get inside the door, clinic escorts are possibly the only source of human connection and visible support that some of these patients and their companions experience. For that moment in time, the human connection supersedes everything. I may vote differently than the patients I serve. They may be deeply religious, while I'm not. We might love rival sports teams. Whatever. The relationship between the clinic escort and the patient bypasses these superficial divisions. It's about a fundamental human need to be seen and valued, particularly in the face of cruelty. It's about human dignity. It's about humanity.

Abortion is, at its core, about life, just not in the way that abortion opponents claim. Everything that surrounds getting an abortion—from the decision to the cost to travel and getting in the door—is about someone's life, the course of that life, the value of that life. That's why I never argue about when a "life" begins, because that isn't the point. The life of the pregnant person is the point. The course of their life is the point. The realities and complexities and hardships and accomplishments: they matter. Their actual, embodied life transcends any philosophical debate in that moment, because I can see with my own eyes and feel with my own heart the weight of that life, the importance of that person's ability to determine what happens to their own life.

That is the power of volunteering as a clinic escort at its most fundamental. It reclaims that space and centers the person having the abortion, rather than the people standing in her way. When we replace the face of abortion with a human being, rather than a theoretical or political argument, it becomes clear what to do: support people's lives.

To do that doesn't require a legal degree or a political background. It isn't something that only bullhorn-wielding activists and lobbyists do. It is something that each of us can do, in our own way. Maybe volunteering as a clinic escort isn't something you can do. That's okay. We don't need everyone to do the same job. We just need everyone to do a job. There are so many ways to get involved and support abortion access. Write thank-you notes to abortion providers and clinic staff. Donate to your local abortion fund. Call your legislators and ask them where they stand on abortion rights, and what concrete policies to improve abortion access they're willing to support. Find out if there's an abortion clinic near you, and be aware of the protest activity that happens outside. Write a letter to the editor of your local newspaper about why your state needs an enforceable buffer zone at reproductive health clinics. Or simply say out loud that you support access to safe abortion care.

"Every day that you're out there, you change somebody's life for the better," Paula Harris, a longtime clinic escort in Pittsburgh, Pennsylvania, said to me.[54] What will you do today to change somebody's life for the better?

We all have the power, and the responsibility, to pick up the proverbial vest and do our part. If we do, we can not only end this crisis—we can ensure that it never happens again.

• • •

By 6:00 a.m. on the morning of February 11, 2017, a wall of pink stretched across three sides of the Planned Parenthood clinic in Savannah, Georgia. Fifty people stood, shoulder to shoulder, awaiting the wave of antiabortion protesters that would soon descend on the clinic. Among the crowd was a seventy-three-year-old woman wearing a bright pink T-shirt that read I STAND WITH PLANNED PARENTHOOD in bold white letters. It was Dandy Barrett.

Now a year older than her father James was when he was murdered by an antiabortion terrorist, Barrett hasn't stopped speaking out about abortion rights and antiabortion violence. In the years since his death, she continued to support abortion rights, speaking at events, sharing her father's legacy. But today, she was going to do more than speak.

Some local activists had heard that antiabortion protesters were planning to target Savannah's Planned Parenthood clinic for the day. While this Planned Parenthood didn't even provide abortions, the protesters still planned to show up and make a scene. The activists decided that they would be there too, a wall of protection between the protesters and the clinic entrance. They would position themselves off the property so as not to disturb patients, but they would make sure that protesters couldn't get beyond them to harass anyone.

"They called me and said, 'We're going to be out there at 6:00 a.m., and we're going to ring the establishment so they can't get anywhere near it,'" Barrett recalled.[55] Did she want to join them? She didn't hesitate—she was in.

When the protesters showed up an hour later, it was too late to get near the clinic at all. "We ringed it," Barrett proudly recalled. "They couldn't even try."[56]

It had been nearly a quarter of a century since Paul Hill murdered her father and Dr. Britton. Donald Trump was president of the United States. Hundreds of abortion restrictions had passed in state legislatures across the country. The cause for which her father ultimately gave his life had rapidly regressed before Barrett's eyes.

But not on this day. Not at this clinic. On this day, Dandy Barrett carried with her the legacy of her father and the thousands of others who served as clinic escorts—she put her body on the line to support those who needed reproductive health care.

It was a few hours, at most. The protesters eventually left, and so did Barrett and the other volunteers. She didn't submit a legal challenge to an abortion law by being out there. She didn't alter the course of a potential Supreme Court ruling on *Roe v. Wade*. It was so much smaller than that, and so much bigger. It was kindness and empathy. It was human dignity. It was an act of service. It was what her father did so many years ago. It was the cause for which he gave his life.

How would he feel, seeing her out there, still doing what he did in 1994?

"He would be incredulous that the issue was still an issue. That would have just appalled him . . . And he would have understood that there are people, many people like himself, who would have said, 'By gum, I have to stand up.'"[57]

Epilogue

Hindsight Is 2020

WHEN I FIRST BEGAN CONCEPTUALIZING THIS BOOK IN EARLY
2019, the epilogue was meant to be a reflection on the results of
the 2020 presidential election. The outcome of that race could determine the future of legal abortion in America. At the time, the
election seemed like the most important event that could possibly
happen that year.

But of course, 2020 had other plans.

I began writing this book in earnest in April 2020, a month
into lockdown from the coronavirus pandemic, four months after
moving from New York to Colorado, a month before police officer
Derek Chauvin murdered George Floyd, seven months out from that
pivotal presidential election. In some ways, it helped me focus my
energy. I was able to channel my anxiety and fear into a tangible
project. Scanning through buried archives, digging up old, tattered
newspaper articles, conducting interview after interview—it helped.
I dove into the stories of my fellow clinic escorts while remaining
largely holed up in my home, isolating to protect my partner and
myself from the pandemic. I couldn't volunteer as a clinic escort anymore, but I could try to tell this story, our story, a story of resilience
and fortitude in the face of hostility and hatred.

Joe Biden was finally declared president-elect on November 7, 2020, four days after the polls closed. Spontaneous celebrations burst forth in cities across America. Cheers echoed across my neighborhood. My partner and I hugged, tears gathering in our eyes. I was profoundly relieved, as were so many of us. But the damage of the past four years—of the past four decades—to safe and legal abortion couldn't be undone in a day. It can't be undone by the Biden presidency. It will have to be slowly, systematically undone by all of us.

As the pandemic worsened and the death toll mounted through-out 2020, the story I was writing echoed so much of the turbulence through which we were all living. Whose lives matter? Who is af-forded the ability to exercise their right to bodily autonomy, and who isn't? How responsible are we for each other? Who gets to be "free," and who doesn't?

Wearing a mask, a basic public health protection, became a po-litically charged decision. Many of the same people who publicly pushed for an end to legal abortion, including many Republicans in Congress and antiabortion terrorists like John Brockhoeft, now championed their right to choose what they did with their own bod-ies to avoid wearing masks in public places. Hundreds of thousands of Americans would ultimately die from COVID-19, a dispropor-tionate number of whom were Black.[1]

A white police officer kneeled on the neck of George Floyd, an unarmed Black man, for nearly ten minutes, murdering him in front of a traumatized teenage girl with a camera. Louisville police invaded the home of Breonna Taylor, an unarmed Black woman and an EMT for the city, while she was sleeping and shot and killed her. Those same police officers were never charged with her murder. Nationwide protests erupted in the wake of these and other police killings of Black people. They were met with organized, systematic brutality and violence on the part of law enforcement, from New York to Los Angeles.

These issues may not seem connected to abortion access, but they are. Black lives are subjected to routine brutality, torture, and murder at the hands of those who we also call upon to "protect" abortion providers from threats and aggression. Refusing to wear a mask in a grocery store threatens the health, safety, and security of others, as does trying to block someone from exiting a car in front of an abortion clinic. Bans on gender-affirming care for trans youth, like what Arkansas passed in early 2021, violate our most sacred right to self-determination. So do abortion bans.

All of these issues, as disparate as they may seem, are about our fundamental American values.

Defeating Donald Trump was not only essential to the future of safe and legal abortion, but also to the future of democracy itself. But that defeat was simply a tiny step back from the ledge onto which this country has walked itself, often on the backs of the most marginalized. The next step is up to all of us.

I'm under no illusions that this book will solve the ongoing abortion rights crisis in this country. As I'm writing this now, in September 2021, I'll admit that there are times when it's hard to still feel hopeful. But that's when I come back to the incredible people I feature in this book. When abortion was still illegal in almost every state, Carol Downer didn't just tacitly accept it—she found a way to help people access safe underground abortions. After his clinic was bombed in 1986, Dr. George Tiller hung a sign outside the rubble that read HELL NO, WE WON'T GO![2] Upon hearing that Operation Rescue was heading to Buffalo, New York, to wreak havoc like they did in Wichita, Ellie Dorritie and her compatriots created a massive clinic defense effort that kept every clinic open. And two decades after her father was murdered for volunteering as a clinic escort,

Dandy Barrett stood outside a Planned Parenthood, a defiant display of support in the face of anti-choice hostility.

In June 2020, four months before she died, I spoke to Sue Davis about her time as a clinic escort and defender. She told me about one of the earliest abortion rights rallies she attended in New York in 1970. "I *still* have a button from that demonstration," she said. I asked her why she kept it all these years. "As a reminder," she explained. "I never want to forget what we went through [before *Roe v. Wade*], and what we made happen."

I know that *Roe v. Wade* is finished, but I also know this: The Supreme Court doesn't get to decide what happens to safe abortion. We do.

Acknowledgments

WRITING A BOOK IS NEVER TRULY A SOLITARY ACT. WRITING this book, about the power of community and coming together, truly took a village. It has been an immense honor and privilege to try to tell the story of my fellow clinic escorts and of the unique role that we've played in protecting access to this basic right. I am forever indebted to so many people who have supported me on this journey.

First and foremost, a profound thank you to my editors, Dan Smetanka and Jennifer Alton. Dan immediately knew what this book was trying to be and why this story needed to be told, and he gave me carte blanche permission to do it. Dan and Jennifer were instrumental in bringing my fledgling idea into this full story, and their encouragement and thoughtful guidance made all the differ- ence. And thank you to the entire Counterpoint team for embracing this story and working so hard to help it be told!

This book simply wouldn't have existed if it weren't for my agent Kathy Schneider, who supported me every step of the way in this process. She believed in this book when it didn't even exist yet, and it wouldn't be here, in your hands, without her incredible guidance and encouragement. Thank you to the entire team at Jane Rotrosen Agency for their hard work and support, and a special shout-out to Chris Prestia, who helped connect Kathy and me.

Profound gratitude to each and every person with whom I spoke for this book. To the clinic escorts and defenders: you are the reason for this story, and your fortitude and conviction continue to inspire me. To the activists, clinic owners, and leaders of this movement—you refuse to let this basic right erode without a fight. Endless thanks to you all: Angela Anders, Edmund Cardoni, Erin Clark, Jemal Cole, Michelle Colon, Cory Ellen, Leslie Fillingham, Kimya Forouzan, Kim Gibson, Geoff Green, Derenda Hancock, Helmi Henkin, Laura Horowitz, Becca Howes-Michel, Travis Jackson, Angus Johnston, Julie Magidson, Deirdre Mondel, Karen Musick, Sheila O'Neill, Joel Reese, Jim Sailer, Meg Sasse Stern, Rita Sasse, Paula Schneider, Tamara Soroko, Cara Tenenbaum, Benita Ulisano, Carol Wayman, Aliza Worthington, Andrea Long, Ruth Lednicer, Mary Greenberg, Susan Davis, Kristin Hady, Kay Schwarzwalter, Rachel Borsich, Ashley Gray, Natalie Beach, Shireen Shakouri, Moira Ariev, Emily Goldberg-Hall, Kathryn Ranieri, Heather Mobley, Shelby Greenwell, Nat Cohen, Brittany Meade, Doug Marsh, Yvonne Hilst, Hanna Roe, Barbara Schwartz, Ali Taylor, Jackie Kazarian, Mallory Schwartz, Roxane Sutocky, Alison Dreith, Thomas O'Brian, Carol Hornbeck, Steve Leary, Jonathan McDowell, Linda Kocher, Sue Frietsche, Paula Harris, Autumn Reinhardt-Simpson, Stacey Burns, Liz Gustafson, Michelle Love-Davis, Kerouac Smith, Hilary Ray, Kim Hady, Eleanor Rosenthal, Justine Colom, Ellie Dorritie, Hannah Servedio, Moira Donegan, Bill Friedman, Ann Horn, Mariceli Alegria, Anne Dietz, Bianca Cameron-Schwiesow, Laura Reich, Valerie Peterson, Gretchen McClean, Christine Taylor, Nicole Fonsh, Brittany Conner, Jay Griffin, Jessie Losch, Leila McNeill, Rachel Brown, Lila Baker, Alicia Lucksted, Danielle Lescure, Angela Bocage, Carl Madden, Shanna Atchley-Stafer, Linda Ring, Amanda Ehrhardt, Maddox Pennington, Lindsay Cogan, Gary Lura, James Silvers, Pearl Brady, Becca Ballenger, Robin Frisella, Dianne Mathiowetz, Steph Black, Odile Schalit, Carol Downer, Amy Hagstrom Miller, Tammi

Kromenaker, Calla Hales, Claire Keys, Renee Bracey Sherman, Dandy Barrett, duVergne Gaines, Jeanne Clark, Julie Burkhart, Erin Matson, and so many others in this movement.

This book required a breadth of research, from publicly listed data to buried archives. It couldn't have been done without the following organizations and archival sources: the Guttmacher Institute, the Feminist Majority Foundation, the National Abortion Federation, the Washington Area Clinic Defense Task Force, the BACAOR Clinic Defense Archives, the Adeline Levine Archive at the University of Buffalo, the National Organization for Women Archives, the Schlesinger Library on the History of Women in America at the Harvard Radcliffe Institute, and the Women's Action Coalition Archives at the New York Public Library.

I'm lucky to have an incredible network of personal support, one on which I have called more often than I can count for words of comfort and encouragement. Stephanie Psaki always believed in this book and in me, even when I didn't, and she always nudged me back to self-love by reminding me that this book was "my destiny." Ashley Gray, thank you for showing me what true leadership looks like, for martinis, and for bringing me to clinic escorting in the first place. My dear friend Tamara Drew has never left my corner since I met her more than a decade ago, and she has steadfastly encouraged me to stand in my power and challenge my privilege. And Brittany Tatum, thank you for continually reminding me that I can in fact write, and for being my aesthetic guru (and photographer).

To others who offered me love and support, big and small, in helping me bring this book to life: Sara Pellegrom, Emily Mello, Cecilia Zvosec, Savannah Russo, Kate Bernyk, Aisha Akhter, Jennifer Brunet, Johanna Lindau, Martha Plimpton, Kera Bolonik, Meredith Clair, Catherine Newman, Kellie Overbey, Jenn Lyon, Lecy Goranson, Xorje Olivares, Shannon Harvey, Alison Turkos, Molly

Grodin, Elizabeth Reaser, Rebecca Traister, Dr. Jen Gunter, Adam Frankel, Rachel Friedman, Anna Maltby Patil, Lori Adelman, Lauren Himiak, Eileen Spangler, Emerie Lukas, Lauren Glenn, Sophie Coffey, Sean Coffey, Aubrey Winkler, Ariana DeBose, Katie Dunn, Sarah Vieweg, Amanda Botur, Allie Wittry, Mónica de Pinto Ribeiro Hancke, Katherine Homes, and so many more. You all prove the power of individual acts of kindness and love. Thank you!

To my wonderful family: Thank you for sticking with me and supporting me through this process and everything else. Thank you to my mother and father, Amy and Steve Rankin, who always allowed and encouraged me to pursue my dreams and instilled in me the importance of speaking up against injustice and showing up for those in need. To my brother and sister-in-law, Nick Rankin and Jenna Vondrasek—you both have always cheered me on while finding a way to make me laugh. To Jacki Sharpe and Dominic Latorraca for loving me unconditionally and embodying strength of character. To Beth Wintroub, Tim Schabacker, Sam Schabacker, and Stephanie Lowenthal-Savy for welcoming me into your family with open arms and celebrating my success as your own.

And to my love, Noah Schabacker: When I first interviewed you for this book in the spring of 2019, I had no idea that I was talking to my future husband. We fell in love over the phone, talking about our shared experiences and values, and we have been lucky enough to make a life together. This book brought us together, and I couldn't be more grateful! Thank you for reading every word of this book (twice, sometimes three times), for never losing faith in me or this story, and for showing me the power of love and commitment.

Notes

Preface: So That Happened

1. Kirstein, Marielle, Joerg Dreweke, Rachel K. Jones, and Jesse Philbin. "100 Days Post-Roe: At Least 66 Clinics Across 15 States Have Stopped Offering Abortion Care." Guttmacher Institute. October 2022. www.guttmacher.org/2022/10/100 -days-post-roe-least-66-clinics-across-15-us-states-have -stopped-offering-abortion-care.

Introduction: How Did We Get Here?

1. Mary Ziegler, "The Supreme Court Just Took a Case That Could Kill Roe v. Wade—or Let It Die Slowly," *The Washington Post*, May 18, 2021.

2. Rachel K. Jones, Elizabeth Witwer, Jenna Jerman, "Abortion Incidence and Service Availability in the United States, 2017," Guttmacher Institute, September 2019, accessed May 15, 2021, www.guttmacher.org/report/abortion-incidence-service -availability-us-2017.

3. Terry Gross, "Once Militantly Anti-Abortion, Evangelical Minister Now Lives 'With Regret,'" *Fresh Air*, NPR, July 11, 2018, www.npr.org/2018/07/11/628000131 /once-militantly-anti-abortion-evangelical-minister-now -lives-with-regret.

4. Gross, "Evangelical Minister Now Lives 'With Regret.'"

Chapter One: The Birth of a Movement

1. "Weather History for Rockville, MD, August 2, 1975," *Old Farmer's Almanac*, www.almanac.com/weather/history/MD /Rockville/1975-08-02.

2. Grace Elizabeth Hale, *A Nation of Outsiders: How the White Middle Class Fell in Love with Rebellion in Post-War America* (New York City: Oxford University Press, 2014), 282.

3. Rachel Benson Gold, "Lessons from Before Roe: Will Past be Prologue?" *Guttmacher Policy Review*, Vol. 6, Issue 1 (March 1, 2003), www.guttmacher.org/gpr/2003/03 /lessons-roe-will-past-be-prologue.

4. Phone interview with Carol Downer, May 3, 2019.

5. S. K. Henshaw, J. D. Forrest, E. Sullivan, C. Tietze, "Abortion Services in the United States, 1979 and 1980," *Family Planning Perspectives*, Jan–Feb 1982; 14(1):5-8, 10-15, www.ncbi.nlm.nih .gov/pubmed/7037447.

6. S. K. Henshaw, J. D. Forrest, J. Van Vort, "Abortion services in the United States, 1984 and 1985," *Family Planning Perspectives*, Mar–Apr 1987; 19(2):63–70, pubmed.ncbi.nlm.nih .gov/3595820.

7. Johanna Schoen, *Abortion After Roe* (Chapel Hill: University of North Carolina Press, 2015), 161–162.

8. Schoen, *Abortion After Roe*, 170.

9. Schoen, *Abortion After Roe*, 162.

10. Eleanor Bader and Patricia Baird-Windle, *Targets of Hatred: Anti-Abortion Terrorism* (New York: Palgrave Macmillan Trade, 2001), 53.

11. Stephen Braun, "Abortion's Wary Line of Defense: Volunteers Who Escort Doctors and Patients Fear Increased Danger After the Slayings in Florida. They and Protesters Play a

Cat-and-Mouse Game of Intimidation and Protection," *Los Angeles Times*, Aug 11, 1992, www.latimes.com/archives/la -xpm-1994-08-11-mn-25962-story.html.

12. Schoen, *Abortion After Roe*, 164–165.

13. Schoen, *Abortion After Roe*, 164–165.

14. National Abortion Federation, "2019 Violence and Disruption Statistics," 11, prochoice.org/wp-content/uploads/violence _stats.pdf.

15. Bader and Baird-Windle, *Targets of Hatred*, 64.

16. Bader and Baird-Windle, *Targets of Hatred*, 64–65.

17. Bader and Baird-Windle, *Targets of Hatred*, 64–66.

18. Katherine Taylor, testimony, House Subcommittee on Civil and Constitutional Rights, Hearing, March 6, 1985, www .c-span.org/video/?125348-1/abortion-clinic-violence.

19. Taylor, testimony.

20. Feminist Majority Foundation, "Part II – 1984," feminist.org, accessed April 21, 2020, feminist.org/resources/feminist -chronicles/the-feminist-chronicles-2/part-ii-1984.

21. Linda Witt, "Man with a Mission," *Chicago Tribune*, August 11, 1985, www.chicagotribune.com/news/ct-xpm-1985-08-11 -8502220141-story.html.

22. Bader and Baird-Windle, *Targets of Hatred*, 93.

23. Alissa J. Rubin, "The 'Other' Abortion Case," *The Washington Post*, March 22, 1992.

24. Bader and Baird-Windle, *Targets of Hatred*, 87.

25. Schoen, *Abortion After Roe*, 187.

26. Phone interview with Amy Hagstrom Miller, May 19, 2020.

27. Howard Kurtz, "Operation Rescue Aggressively Anti-abortion," *The Washington Post*, March 6, 1989, www .washingtonpost.com/archive/politics/1989/03/06/operation

-rescue-aggressively-antiabortion/1f6a0302-d2be-4efb-af7d
-66059acc2332.

28. Francis Wilkinson, "The Gospel According to Randall Terry," *Rolling Stone*, October 5, 1989, www.rollingstone.com/culture /culture-news/the-gospel-according-to-randall-terry-47951.

29. Phone interview with Susan Davis, April 29, 2020.

30. Faye Ginsburg, "Rescuing the Nation," *Abortion Wars: A Half Century of Struggle, 1950–2000*, ed. Rickie Solinger (Berkeley: University of California Press, 1998), 227.

31. Sheldon Ekland-Olsen, *Who Lives, Who Dies, Who Decides?: Abortion, Neonatal Care, Assisted Dying, and Capital Punishment* (Routledge, 2011), 162.

32. Schoen, *Abortion After Roe*, 188.

33. Wilkinson, "The Gospel According to Randall Terry."

34. Chauncey Bailey and Robert Ourlian, "Abortion Groups Face Off at Clinic," *Detroit News*, September 20, 1987.

35. Schoen, *Abortion After Roe*, 191.

36. Scott H. Ainsworth and Brian M. Harward, *Political Groups, Parties, and Organizations that Shaped America: An Encyclopedia and Document Collection* (ABC-CLIO, 2019), 741–743.

37. Schoen, *Abortion After Roe*, 192.

38. Schoen, *Abortion After Roe*, 187.

39. Phone interview with Dianne Mathiowetz, June 9, 2020.

40. Schoen, *Abortion After Roe*, 193

41. Kurtz, "Operation Rescue Aggressively Antiabortion."

42. Warren Hern, "Life on the Front Lines," in *Abortion Wars: A Half Century of Struggle*, ed. Rickie Solinger (Berkeley: University of California Press, 1998), 313–314.

43. Lisa Myers, "Supreme Court/Abortion/Federal Judge," *NBC Nightly News*, October 16, 1991, tvnews.vanderbilt.edu /programs/578043.

44. Schoen, *Abortion After Roe*, 194.

45. Bay Area Coalition Against Operation Rescue, "We Won't Go Back," 1989, archive.org/details/abortrts.

46. Bay Area Coalition Against Operation Rescue, "BACAOR Clinic Defense: A Model," brochure, January 1, 1990, archive .org/details/BACAORClinicDefenseAModel/page/n5 /mode/2up.

47. Phone interview with Angela Bocage, May 28, 2020.

48. "BACAOR Clinic Defense: A Model."

49. "BACAOR Clinic Defense: A Model."

50. Jo Freeman and Victoria Johnson, *Waves of Protest: Social Movements Since the Sixties* (Lanham, MD: Rowman & Littlefield Publishers, 1999), 247–248.

51. Phone interview with Alicia Lucksted, May 26, 2020.

52. Associated Press Staff, "More Than 350 Arrested in Abortion Protests in 5 States," Associated Press, January 28, 1989, apnews.com/64d8617c99bdf915b78d2e7bd8ea9cc0.

53. "More Than 350 Arrested in Abortion Protests in 5 States."

54. Phone interview with Danielle Lescure, May 28, 2020.

55. New York Pro-Choice Coalition, "The Battle to Defend Abortion Clinics: Organizing Against 'Operation Rescue,'" www.merlehoffman.com/wp-content/uploads/2017/02 /MerlePamphlet_singlePDF.pdf.

56. Phone interview with Mary Lou Greenberg, April 29, 2020.

57. "The Battle to Defend Abortion Clinics: Organizing Against 'Operation Rescue.'"

58. Greenberg, interview.

59. Rodney P. Carlisle, *Encyclopedia of Politics: The Left and the Right*, Vol. 1 (Thousand Oaks, CA: SAGE Publications, 2005), 518.

60. "The Battle to Defend Abortion Clinics: Organizing Against 'Operation Rescue.'"

61. "George Tiller Timeline," *The Wichita Eagle,* March 1, 2011, www.kansas.com/news/special-reports/article1007186.html.

62. Bader and Baird-Windle, *Targets of Hatred,* 158.

63. Marty Cohen, *Moral Victories in the Battle for Congress: Cultural Conservatism and the House GOP* (Philadelphia: University of Pennsylvania Press, 2019), 75.

64. Jennifer Donnally, "Summer of Mercy," *Kansas History: A Journal of the Central Plains* 39 (Winter 2016–2017): 259, www.kshs.org/publicat/history/2016winter_donnally.pdf.

65. Phone interview with Julie Burkhart, June 1, 2020.

66. Wichita Public Radio, "Operation Rescue 1991," December 12, 2014, YouTube video, www.youtube.com/watch?v=NjbJb7Tal1M.

67. *Clinic Blockades: Hearing Before the Subcommittee on Crime and Criminal Justice of the Committee on the Judiciary,* 102nd Cong., Second Session, May 6, 1992, play.google.com/books/reader?id=Y8UllRiN8QUC&hl=en&pg=GBS.PA15 Page 14.

68. Testimony from Sylvia Doe, House Subcommittee on Crime and Criminal Justice, 102nd Cong., Second Session, May 6, 1992.

69. Testimony, Sylvia Doe.

70. Wichita Public Radio, "Operation Rescue 1991."

71. Wichita Public Radio, "Operation Rescue 1991."

72. Don Terry, "As the Nation Debate Abortion, A Judge Is Cast as the Moderator," *The New York Times,* August 9, 1991, www.nytimes.com/1991/08/09/us/as-the-nation-debates-abortion-a-judge-is-cast-as-the-moderator.html.

73. Carol Mason, *Killing for Life: The Apocalyptic Narrative of Pro-Life Politics* (Ithaca, NY: Cornell University Press, 2002), 102.

74. Cohen, *Moral Victories in the Battle for Congress,* 75.

75. Jim McLean, "My Fellow Kansans: The Summer of Mercy," NPR, September 24, 2018, www.kbia.org/post/my-fellow -kansans-summer-mercy#stream/0.

76. Sabra Moore, *Openings: A Memoir from the Women's Art Movement, New York City 1970–1992* (New York: New Village Press, 2016), 364.

77. Phone interview with Ellie Dorritie, May 14, 2020.

78. Mathiowetz, interview.

79. Mary B. W. Tabor, "Buffalo Braces for Renewal of Abortion Protests," *The New York Times*, March 7, 1992, www .nytimes.com/1992/03/07/nyregion/buffalo-braces-for -renewal-of-abortion-protests.html.

80. Catherine S. Manegold, "Protests in Buffalo Fade Into a Footnote to Abortion," *The New York Times*, May 3, 1992, www .nytimes.com/1992/05/03/nyregion/protests-in-buffalo-fade -into-a-footnote-to-abortion.html.

81. National Commission on America Without Roe, *Facing a Future Without Choice—A Report on Reproductive Liberty in America* (Washington, D.C.: NARAL Foundation, 1992).

82. Linda Feldmann, "Anti-Abortion Group Hits Buffalo, but with New Tactics," *Christian Science Monitor*, April 22, 1992, www.csmonitor.com/1992/0422/22092.html.

83. Bader and Baird-Windle, *Targets of Hatred*, 174.

84. Dorritie, interview.

85. Dorritie, interview.

86. Dorritie, interview.

87. Bader and Baird-Windle, *Targets of Hatred*, 174.

88. Dorritie, interview.

89. Mathiowetz, interview.

90. Phone interview with Ann Horn, May 15, 2020.

91. Greenberg, interview.

92. Phone interview with Susan Davis, April 29, 2020.

93. Bader and Baird-Windle, *Targets of Hatred*, 174.

94. Dorritie, interview.

95. Horn, interview.

96. "Police Arrest 190 in Anti-abortion Demonstration," UPI, April 22, 1992, www.upi.com/Archives/1992/04/22/Police-arrest-190-in-anti-abortion-demonstration/5749703915200.

97. Mathiowetz, interview.

98. Dorritie, interview.

99. Catherine S. Manegold, "Abortion War, Buffalo Front: Top Guns Use Battle Tactics," *The New York Times*, April 25, 1992, www.nytimes.com/1992/04/25/nyregion/abortion-war-buffalo-front-top-guns-use-battle-tactics.html.

100. Gene Warner, "Spring of Life Fails to Live Up to the Hype Yet Effort Puts Issue in Spotlight," *Buffalo News*, May 3, 1992, buffalonews.com/1992/05/03/spring-of-life-fails-to-live-up-to-hype-yet-effort-puts-issue-in-spotlight.

101. "Police Arrest 190 in Anti-Abortion Demonstration."

102. Priscilla Painton, "Buffalo Operation Fizzle," *Time*, May 4, 1992, content.time.com/time/magazine/article/0,9171,975413,00.html.

103. "Women's Issues: NOW National Press Briefing," C-SPAN, June 12, 1992, www.c-span.org/video/?26553-1/womens-issues.

104. Phone interview with Moira Ariev, April 29, 2020.

105. National Abortion Federation, "2019 Violence and Disruption Statistics Report."

106. Phone interview with Jeanne Clark, May 24, 2020.

107. Horn, interview.

Chapter Two: I Fought the Law and the Law Won

1. Phone interview with Dandy Barrett, May 2020.

2. Barrett, interview, May 2020.

3. Sara Rimer, "The Clinic Gunman and the Victim: Abortion Fight Reflected in 2 Lives," *The New York Times*, March 14, 1993, www.nytimes.com/1993/03/14/us/the-clinic-gunman -and-the-victim-abortion-fight-reflected-in-2-lives.html.

4. Barrett, interview, June 2019.

5. Sam Howe Verhovek, "Slain Clinic Escort Saw Job as a Mission," *The New York Times*, August 5, 1994, www.nytimes .com/1994/08/05/us/slain-clinic-escort-saw-job-as-a-mission .html.

6. "Weather History for Pensacola, FL, July 29, 1994," *Old Farmer's Almanac*, www.almanac.com/weather/history/FL /Pensacola/1994-07-29.

7. Wilkinson, "The Gospel According to Randall Terry."

8. *Abortion Clinic Violence: Hearing Before the Subcommittee on Crime and Criminal Justice on the Committee of the Judiciary*, 103rd Cong., First Section, April 1, 1993.

9. *Abortion Clinic Violence: Hearing Before the Subcommittee on Crime and Criminal Justice on the Committee of the Judiciary*, 103rd Cong., First Section, June 10, 1993, 191.

10. Phone interview with Anne G., June 5, 2020.

11. *Clinic Blockades: Hearing Before the Subcommittee on Crime and Criminal Justice of the Committee on the Judiciary*, 102nd Cong., Second Session, May 6, 1992.

12. *Clinic Blockades: Hearing Before the Subcommittee on Crime and Criminal Justice of the Committee on the Judiciary*, 102nd Cong., Second Session, May 6, 1992.

13. State of Wis. v. Missionaries to the Preborn, 796 F. Supp. 389

(E.D. Wis. 1992), law.justia.com/cases/federal/district-courts /FSupp/796/389/1559206.

14. "Operation Rescue Activists Resist Abortion Clinic in Wichita, Kansas (Summer of Mercy), 1991," Global Nonviolent Action Database, nvdatabase.swarthmore.edu/content/operation-rescue -activists-resist-abortion-clinic-wichita-kansas-summer -mercy-1991.

15. Freedom of Access to Clinic Entrances Act, Pub. L. No. 103-259, 108 Stat. 694) (May 26, 1994, 18 U.S.C. § 248), www .govtrack.us/congress/bills/103/s636.

16. Freedom of Access to Clinic Entrances Act.

17. "Abortion Clinic Access Bill Signing," C-SPAN, May 26, 1994, www.c-span.org/video/?57299-1/abortion-clinic-access-bill -signing.

18. Bader and Baird-Windle, *Targets of Hatred*, 128.

19. Bader and Baird-Windle, *Targets of Hatred*, 147.

20. Phone interview with Laura Horowitz, April 12, 2019.

21. Horowitz, interview.

22. Phone interview with Claire Keyes, April 28, 2019.

23. Phone interview with Julie Madison, March 2019.

24. Feminist Majority Foundation, "Monitoring Clinic Violence," feminist.org, accessed June 14, 2020, www.feminist .org/research/cvsurveys/cvsurv_index.html.

25. United States General Accounting Office, Report to the Ranking Minority Member, Subcommittee on Crime, Committee on the Judiciary, House of Representatives, "Abortion Clinics: Information on the Effectiveness of the Freedom of Access to Clinic Entrances Act," November 1998, 44, play .google.com/books/reader?id=RplePoAtODcC&hl=en &pg=GBS.PA44.

26. "Abortion Clinics: Information on the Effectiveness of the Free-
     dom of Access to Clinic Entrances Act," November 1998, 60–61,
     play.google.com/books/reader?id=RplePoAtODcC&hl=en
     &pg=GBS.PA61.

27. Phone interview with Susan Frietsche, May 8, 2020.

28. Lucksted, interview.

29. Brookline Clinic Escorts, "Clinic Escorting Guide," 1996,
     planet4589.org/jcm/politics/ab/public/escort96.txt.

30. Lucksted, interview.

31. Lucksted, interview.

32. Phone interview with Anne G., May 8, 2020.

33. "Abortion Clinics: Information on the Effectiveness of the
     Freedom of Access to Clinic Entrances Act," November
     1998, 41.

34. Phone interview with Jonathan McDowell, May 7, 2020.

35. McDowell, interview.

36. Bader and Baird-Windle, *Targets of Hatred*, 244.

37. McDowell, interview.

38. Phone interview with Leslie Fillingham, April 21, 2019.

39. Keyes, interview.

40. Keyes, interview.

41. Horowitz, interview.

42. Horowitz, interview.

43. Phone interview with Laura Horowitz, April 24, 2020.

44. "Abortion Clinics: Information on the Effectiveness of the
     Freedom of Access to Clinic Entrances Act," November
     1998, 41.

45. Horn, interview.

46. "Neighborhood Report: Out in Front; Through the Eyes
     of Clinic Escorts," *The New York Times*, April 30, 1995,

www.nytimes.com/1995/04/30/nyregion/neighborhood-report
-out-in-front-through-the-eyes-of-clinic-escorts.html.

47. Schoen, *Abortion After Roe*, 172.

48. Schoen, *Abortion After Roe*, 173.

49. Schoen, *Abortion After Roe*, 173.

50. Phone interview with Shanna Atchley-Shafer, June 1, 2020.

51. Phone interview with Benita Ulisano, April 27, 2020.

52. Dorritie, interview.

53. Jim Yardley and David Rohde, "Abortion Doctor in Buffalo
     Slain; Sniper Attack Fits Violent Pattern," *The New York Times*,
     October 25, 1998, www.nytimes.com/1998/10/25/nyregion
     /abortion-doctor-in-buffalo-slain-sniper-attack-fits-violent
     -pattern.html.

54. Bader and Baird-Windle, *Targets of Hatred*, 315.

55. David W. Chen, "A Week of Abortion Protests in Buffalo Be-
     gins Loudly but Peacefully," *The New York Times*, April 19, 1999,
     www.nytimes.com/1999/04/19/nyregion/a-week-of-abortion
     -protests-in-buffalo-begins-loudly-but-peacefully.html.

56. "Weather History for Buffalo, NY, April 20, 1999," *Old
     Farmer's Almanac*, www.almanac.com/weather/history/NY
     /Buffalo/1999-04-20.

57. Lawrence B. Finer, Stanley K. Henshaw, "Abortion Inci-
     dence and Services in the United States in 2000," *Perspectives
     on Sexual and Reproductive Health*, January/February 2003,
     Vol. 35, Issue 1, www.guttmacher.org/journals/psrh/2003/01
     /abortion-incidence-and-services-united-states-2000.

58. Carol Mason, *Killing for Life: The Apocalyptic Narrative of Pro-
     Life Politics* (Ithaca, NY: Cornell University Press, 2002), 101.

59. Dorritie, interview.

60. Roberto Suro, "The Papal Visit; Pope Condemns Abortion
     in U.S. as He Ends Visit," *The New York Times*, September 20,

1987, www.nytimes.com/1987/09/20/us/the-papal-visit-pope
-condemns-abortion-in-us-as-he-ends-visit.html.

61. Fillingham, interview.

62. Barrett, interview, June 2019.

63. Bader and Baird-Windle, *Targets of Hatred*, 229.

64. James Risen, "Suspect Extolled 'Justifiable Homicide' 2 Slain Outside Fla. Abortion Clinic," *The Baltimore Sun*, July 30, 1994, www.baltimoresun.com/news/bs-xpm-1994-07-30-19942 11001-story.html.

65. Schoen, *Abortion After Roe*, 217.

Chapter Three: Too Many to Count

1. Phone interview with Cory Ellen, April 2019.

2. Brian Pendleton, "The California Therapeutic Abortion Act: An Analysis," *Hastings Law Journal*, Vol. 19, Issue 1 (November 1967), Article 11, repository.uchastings.edu/cgi/viewcontent .cgi?article=1968&context=hastings_law_journal.

3. Downer, interview.

4. Feminist Majority Foundation, "National Clinic Access Project," feminist.org, accessed July 1, 2020, feminist.org /our-work/national-clinic-access-project.

5. "In the Courts: Federal Judge Rules California Abortion Clinic 'Bubble' Law Constitutional," National Partnership for Women & Families, August 6, 2009, go.nationalpartnership .org/site/News2?abbr=daily2_&page=NewsArticle&id= 19005.

6. Reihan Salam, "The Worst Ideas of the Decade: Compassion-ate Conservatism," *The Washington Post*, accessed June 24, 2020, www.washingtonpost.com/wp-srv/special/opinions/outlook /worst-ideas/compassionate-conservatism.html.

7. Partial-Birth Abortion Ban Act of 2003, 18 U.S.C. 1531,

November 3, 2003, www.congress.gov/bill/108th-congress /senate-bill/3.

8. Cynthia Dailard, "Courts Strike 'Partial Birth' Abortion Ban; Decisions Presage Future Debates," *Guttmacher Policy Review*, Vol. 7, Issue 4, November 3, 2004, www.guttmacher.org/gpr /2004/11/courts-strike-partial-birth-abortion-ban-decisions -presage-future-debates.

9. Pew Research Center, "The High Court Upholds the Federal Partial Birth Abortion Ban Act," June 6, 2007, www .pewforum.org/2007/06/06/the-high-court-upholds-the -federal-partial-birth-abortion-ban-act.

10. Allyson Chiu, "'Juno' tackled teen pregnancy and abortion. The woman behind the film says she wouldn't write it today," *The Washington Post*, May 17, 2019, www.washingtonpost .com/nation/2019/05/17/juno-diablo-cody-georgia-alabama -abortion-bans.

11. Phone interview with Amy Hagstrom Miller, May 18, 2020.

12. Ulisano, interview, May 3, 2019.

13. Ulisano, interview, April 24, 2020.

14. Alesha Doan, *Opposition and Intimidation: The Abortion Wars and Strategies of Political Harassment* (Ann Arbor: University of Michigan Press, 2007), 1–3.

15. Doan, *Opposition and Intimidation*, 182.

16. "Helping to End the Injustice of Abortion," 40 Days for Life, accessed July 7, 2020. www.40daysforlife.com/about-overview .aspx.

17. Ulisano, interview, April 24, 2020.

18. Ulisano, interview, July 22, 2020.

19. Ulisano, interview, July 22, 2020.

20. United States Court of Appeals for the Seventh Circuit, Veronica Price, et al. v. City of Chicago, et al., No. 16-cv-8268, February

2019, www.supremecourt.gov/DocketPDF/18/18-1516/97765 /20190426142534810_SeventhCirc.pdf.

21. "40 Days for Life," *The Concordian*, October 7, 2010, thecon cordian.org/2010/10/07/40-days-for-life.

22. Erik Eckholm and Kim Severson, "Virginia Senate Passes Ultrasound Bill as Other States Take Notice," *The New York Times,* February 28, 2012, www.nytimes.com/2012/02/29 /us/virginia-senate-passes-revised-ultrasound-bill.html.

23. Jon Stewart, "Punanny State—Virginia's Transvaginal Ultra-sound Bill," *The Daily Show with Jon Stewart*, Comedy Cen-tral, February 21, 2012, www.cc.com/video-clips/83xa8q/the -daily-show-with-jon-stewart-punanny-state---virginia-s -transvaginal-ultrasound-bill.

24. Phone interview with Autumn Reinhardt-Simpson, July 17, 2020.

25. Reinhardt-Simpson, interview.

26. Lucy Madison, "Virginia Gov. Bob McDonnell signs Vir-ginia ultrasound bill," *CBS News*, March 7, 2012, www .cbsnews.com/news/virginia-gov-bob-mcdonnell-signs -virginia-ultrasound-bill.

27. "Helping to End the Injustice of Abortion," 40 Days for Life.

28. National Abortion Federation, "2019 Violence and Disruption Statistics Report."

29. Ulisano, interview, July 22, 2020.

30. Ulisano, interview, July 22, 2020.

31. Interview with Jemal Cole, February 2019.

32. Tara Isabella Burton, "The March for Life, Ameri-ca's biggest anti-abortion rally, explained," *Vox*, January 18, 2018, www.vox.com/identities/2018/1/18/16870018 /march-for-life-anti-abortion-rally-explained.

33. "Weather History for Charlotte, NC, November 9, 2016," *Old*

Farmer's Almanac, www.almanac.com/weather/history/NC /Charlotte/2016-11-09.

34. Phone interview with Laura Reich, May 19, 2020.

35. Phone interview with Angela Anders, 2019.

36. Jenavieve Hatch, "North Carolina Abortion Providers Fight for Ground amid Growing Hostility," *HuffPost,* December 4, 2016, www.huffpost.com/entry/charlotte-abortion-rights -protest_n_5841b859e4b0c68e04808b82.

37. Anders, interview.

38. Lindsay Beyerstein and Martyna Starosta, "Care in Chaos," 2017, Vimeo via Rewire News Group, rewirenewsgroup.com /videos/2017/07/11/care-in-chaos.

39. Phone interview with Rachel Borsich, April 27, 2020.

40. Phone interview with Heather Mobley, April 30, 2020.

41. Reich, interview.

42. Phone interview with Calla Hales, May 28, 2020.

43. Ryan Pitkin, "A Movement Grows Outside of East Charlotte Abortion Clinic," *Queen City Nerve,* September 24, 2020, qcnerve.com/new-defenders-charlotte-abortion-clinic.

44. Phone interview with Hanna Roze, May 5, 2020.

45. Ulisano, interview, July 22, 2020.

46. Ulisano, interview, April 2019.

47. Ulisano, interview, July 22, 2020.

48. Ulisano, interview, July 22, 2020.

49. Ulisano, interview, July 22, 2020.

50. Mobley, interview.

51. Beyerstein and Starosta, "Care in Chaos."

52. Mobley, interview.

53. Beyerstein and Starosta, "Care in Chaos."

54. Hales, interview.

55. Phone interview with Cory Ellen, February 2019.

56. Interview with Natalie Beach, April 28, 2020.

Chapter Four: Last Clinic Standing

1. "State Facts About Abortion: Texas," Guttmacher Institute, last updated January 2021, www.guttmacher.org/fact-sheet /state-facts-about-abortion-texas.

2. Amy Hagstrom Miller, "SCOTUS Abortion-Rights Plaintiff: Texas Win Is Just the Start," *Time*, June 27, 2016, time .com/4384022/supreme-court-abortion-ruling-plaintiff.

3. "Plaintiff Reaction to Supreme Court Ruling on Texas Abortion Restrictions," C-SPAN, June 27, 2016, www.c-span.org /video/?411779-103/plaintiff-reaction-supreme-court-ruling -texas-abortion-restrictions.

4. "Plaintiff Reaction to Supreme Court Ruling on Texas Abortion Restrictions."

5. "Targeted Regulation of Abortion Providers," Guttmacher Institute, last updated June 1, 2021, www.guttmacher.org /state-policy/explore/targeted-regulation-abortion-providers.

6. "Communities Need Clinics 2019 Report: Independent Abortion Care Providers and the Landscape of Abortion Care in the United States," Abortion Care Network, 7-9, abortioncarenetwork.org/wp-content/uploads/2020/08 /CommunitiesNeedClinics2019.pdf.

7. "Peristats: Birth Rate in Texas, 2009–2019," March of Dimes, accessed August 2, 2020, www.marchofdimes.org/peristats /presentations/brthrate_TX_2009_2019_grph_1_r534.pdf.

8. Rachel K. Jones, Elizabeth Witwer, Jenna Jerman, "Abortion Incidence and Service Availability in the United States, 2017," September 2019, www.guttmacher.org/report /abortion-incidence-service-availability-us-2017.

9. "QuickFacts: Fargo city, North Dakota," United States

Census, accessed August 8, 2020, www.census.gov/quickfacts/fargocitynorthdakota.

10. Phone interview with Hilary Ray, May 13, 2020.

11. Phone interview with Tammi Kromenaker, April 30, 2020.

12. Reuters Staff, "Federal Judge Strikes Down North Dakota 'Heartbeat' Abortion Law," Reuters, April 16, 2014, www.reuters.com/article/usa-abortion-northdakota/federal-judge-strikes-down-north-dakota-heartbeat-abortion-law-idUSL2N0N81BJ20140416.

13. Nathalie Baptiste, "Anti-Choice 'Personhood' Measures Fail in North Dakota and Colorado," *American Prospect*, November 5, 2014, prospect.org/power/anti-choice-personhood-measures-fail-north-dakota-colorado.

14. Kromenaker, interview.

15. "Bishop Aquila Prays at North Dakota Abortion Clinic as 40 Days for Life Continues," *Catholic News Agency*, September 26, 2009, www.catholicnewsagency.com/news/17228/bishop-aquila-prays-at-north-dakota-abortion-clinic-as-40-days-for-life-continues.

16. Phone interview with Kay Schwarzwalter, April 24, 2020.

17. Kromenaker, interview.

18. Phone interview with Gary Lura, August 8, 2020.

19. Lura, interview.

20. John Eligon and Erik Eckholm, "New Laws Ban Most Abortions in North Dakota," *The New York Times*, March 26, 2013, www.nytimes.com/2013/03/27/us/north-dakota-governor-signs-strict-abortion-limits.html.

21. Associated Press, "North Dakota: Abortion Ban at 6 Weeks Is Overturned," *The New York Times*, April 16, 2014, www.nytimes.com/2014/04/17/us/north-dakota-abortion-ban-at-6-weeks-is-overturned.html.

22. Patrick Springer, "N.D. Abortion Clinic Drops Suit Challenging Law After Reaching Deal with State, March 14, 2014, www.grandforksherald.com/news/2466082-nd-abortion-clinic-drops-suit-challenging-law-after-reaching-deal.

23. Phone interview with Paula Schneider, April 2019.

24. Anna Werner, "Right to Protest Heats Up Outside Kentucky's Last Abortion Clinic," *CBS News*, July 24, 2017, www.cbsnews.com/news/kentucky-abortion-clinic-protest-operation-save-america-buffer-zone.

25. Jessica Arons, "The Last Clinics Standing," ACLU, accessed August 11, 2020, www.aclu.org/issues/reproductive-freedom/abortion/last-clinics-standing.

26. Interview with Rita Sasse, April 30, 2020.

27. Matt Flegenheimer and Maggie Haberman, "Donald Trump, Abortion Foe, Eyes 'Punishment' for Women, Then Recants," *The New York Times*, March 30, 2016, www.nytimes.com/2016/03/31/us/politics/donald-trump-abortion.html.

28. Phone interview with Meg Sasse Stern, April 15, 2019.

29. Phone interview with Erin Clark, November 15, 2019.

30. Madeleine Weiner and Darla Carter, "11 Arrests Made in Protest at Louisville Abortion Clinic in May," *Courier Journal*, May 13, 2017, www.courier-journal.com/story/news/local/2017/05/13/arrests-made-protest-louisville-abortion-clinic-saturday/321109001.

31. Erin Clark, interview.

32. Erin Clark, interview.

33. Sasse Stern, interview.

34. Weiner and Carter, "11 Arrests Made in Protest at Louisville Abortion Clinic in May."

35. Weiner and Carter, "11 Arrests Made in Protest at Louisville Abortion Clinic in May."

36. Schneider, interview.

37. Senait Gebregiorgis and Will Weible, "Pro-choice Advocates Protest Strict Abortion Laws Sweeping Country," WHAS11, May 21, 2019, www.whas11.com/article/news/local/pro-choice -advocates-protest-strict-abortion-laws-sweeping-country /417-dee5d847-3115-4f8c-9308-18e1d4459284.

38. Ryland Barton, "Ky. Legislature Passes Ban on Abortions After Sixth Week of Pregnancy," WVXU, March 15, 2019, www.wvxu.org/post/ky-legislature-passes-ban-abortions -after-sixth-week-pregnancy#stream/0.

39. Sarah Mervosh, "Judge Blocks Kentucky Fetal Heartbeat Law That Bans Abortion After 6 Weeks," *The New York Times,* March 16, 2019, www.nytimes.com/2019/03/16/us/kentucky -fetal-heartbeat-abortion-law.html.

40. Caroline Kelly, "Block on Mississippi's fetal-heartbeat abortion bill is upheld," CNN, February 20, 2020, www .cnn.com/2020/02/20/politics/abortion-mississippi -heartbeat-bill-blocked-circuit-court/index.html.

41. Phone interview with Michelle Colon, August 8, 2019.

42. Shanoor Seervai, "Mississippi's Only Abortion Clinic Gets Renewed Hope after Supreme Court Decision," *STAT News,* July 1, 2016, www.statnews.com/2016/07/01 /mississippi-abortion-clinic.

43. Frank Newport, "Mississippi Retains Standing as Most Religious State," *Gallup,* February 8, 2017, news.gallup.com /poll/203747/mississippi-retains-standing-religious-state.aspx.

44. "Religious Landscape Study: Views About Abortion by State (2014)," Pew Research Center, www.pewforum.org/religious -landscape-study/compare/views-about-abortion/by/state.

45. "State Facts About Abortion: Mississippi," Guttmacher

Institute, last updated June 1, 2021, www.guttmacher.org /fact-sheet/state-facts-about-abortion-mississippi.

46. Rachel Benson Gold, "TRAP Laws Gain Political Traction While Abortion Clinics—and the Women They Serve—Pay the Price," *Guttmacher Policy Review*, Vol. 16, Issue 2, June 25, 2013, www.guttmacher.org/gpr/2013/06/trap-laws-gain -political-traction-while-abortion-clinics-and-women-they -serve-pay-price.

47. Associated Press Staff, "Mississippi Bans Most Abortions After 15 Weeks," *Clarion Ledger*, March 19, 2018, www .clarionledger.com/story/news/politics/2018/03/19 /mississippi-bans-most-abortions-after-15-weeks/440162002.

48. "State Facts About Abortion: Mississippi," Guttmacher Institute, last updated June 1, 2021, www.guttmacher.org/fact-sheet /state-facts-about-abortion-mississippi.

49. "State Report: Mississippi 2020," Talk Poverty, talkpoverty .org/state-year-report/mississippi-2020-report.

50. "State Report: Mississippi 2018," Talk Poverty, talkpoverty .org/state-year-report/mississippi-2018-report.

51. "Overview of Mississippi," *US News and World Report*, accessed August 22, 2020, www.usnews.com/news/best-states /mississippi.

52. "Mississippi Maternal Mortality Report 2013–2016," Mississippi Department of Health, 11–13, msdh.ms.gov/msdhsite /_static/resources/8127.pdf.

53. Phone interview with Derenda Hancock, November 22, 2019.

54. June Medical Services L.L.C. et al v. Russo, Interim Secretary, Louisiana Department of Health and Hospitals," No. 18-1323, June 29, 2020, www.supremecourt.gov/opinions /19pdf/18-1323_c07d.pdf.

55. Hagstrom Miller, interview, May 18, 2020.

56. Kromenaker, interview.

Chapter Five: From Bombs to Bans

1. Andrew Yeager, "Protesters March to Oppose Abortion Ban," WBHM, May 20, 2019 wbhm.org/feature/2019/protesters-march-to-oppose-new-abortion-ban.

2. Phone interview with Tamara Soroko, March 24, 2019.

3. Bader and Baird-Windle, *Targets of Hatred*, 299.

4. Carole Joffe, *Dispatches from the Abortion Wars: The Costs of Fanaticism to Doctors, Patients, and the Rest of Us* (Boston: Beacon Press, 2009), 50.

5. Joe Sutton, "Alabama Again Denies Application of Would-Be Abortion Clinic Operator," CNN, September 13, 2012, www.cnn.com/2012/09/12/us/alabama-abortion-clinic/index.html.

6. Elizabeth Nash, Lizamarie Mohammed, Olivia Cappello, Sophia Naide, "State Policy Trends 2019: A Wave of Abortion Bans, but Some States Are Fighting Back," Guttmacher Institute, December 2019, www.guttmacher.org/article/2019/12/state-policy-trends-2019-wave-abortion-bans-some-states-are-fighting-back.

7. Karen Kasler, Andy Chow, and Jo Ingles, "DeWine Issues 'Stay At Home' Order, Exempting Essential Businesses," *Statehouse News Bureau*, March 22, 2020, www.statenews.org/post/dewine-issues-stay-home-order-exempting-essential-businesses.

8. Melanie Payne, "Facebook Fact Check: Convicted 1980s Abortion Clinic Bomber Attended Ohio Statehouse Protests of Stay-at-Home Order," *Columbus Dispatch*, May 11, 2020, www.dispatch.com/story/news/politics/2020/05/11/facebook-fact-check-convicted-1980s/1217535007.

9.   "Firebomber Gets Strict Parole Rules," *Deseret News*, January 19, 1995, www.deseret.com/1995/1/19/19154403/firebomber -gets-strict-parole-rules.

10.   "Around the Nation; 2 Abortion Clinics Attacked in Cincinnati," *The New York Times*, December 31, 1985, www.nytimes .com/1985/12/31/us/around-the-nation-2-abortion-clinics -attacked-in-cincinnati.html.

11.   Associated Press Staff, "Abortion Clinic Bomber Sentenced," Associated Press, January 11, 1991, apnews.com /article/945283fedfb3ba9c3231f6c098d42cc1.

12.   Jeffrey Kaplan, *Radical Religion and Violence: Theory and Case Studies* (New York: Routledge Press, 2015), 825–826.

13.   Gabe Rosenberg, "A Bill Banning Most Abortions Becomes Law in Ohio," NPR, April 11, 2019, www.npr .org/2019/04/11/712455980/a-bill-banning-most-abortions -becomes-law-in-ohio.

14.   Jason Morton, "Clinic attack suspect has no record of violence," *Tuscaloosanews.com*, April 28, 2006, www.tuscaloosanews .com/article/DA/20060428/News/606114007/TL.

15.   Phone interview with Helmi Henkin, September 1, 2019.

16.   "Past Weather in Tuscaloosa, Alabama: May 2019 Weather in Tuscaloosa," *Timeanddate.com*, www.timeanddate.com /weather/usa/tuscaloosa/historic?month=5&year=2019.

17.   Henkin, interview.

18.   Jamie "JJ" Johnson, "I'm a Clinic Escort in Alabama and I've Been Subject to Harassment and Physical Violence," *Huffpost*, May 21, 2019, www.huffpost.com/entry/abortion-clinic-escort -alabama_n_5ce2c985e4b087700992a282.

19.   Henkin, interview.

20.   Auditi Guha, "In Alabama, an Anti-Choice Protester Tried to Run Over an Abortion Clinic Escort," Rewire News Group,

May 8, 2019, rewirenewsgroup.com/article/2019/05/08/in
-alabama-an-anti-choice-protester-tried-to-run-over-an
-abortion-clinic-escort.

21. Henkin, interview.

22. Johnson, "I'm a Clinic Escort in Alabama."

23. Kate Smith, "Alabama's Near-Total Abortion Ban Blocked by
Federal Judge," *CBS News,* October 29, 2019, www.cbsnews
.com/news/alabama-abortion-law-federal-judge-blocks-near
-total-abortion-ban-from-taking-effect-today-2019-10-29.

24. Henkin, interview.

25. "State Facts About Abortion: Ohio," Guttmacher Institute,
last updated January 2021, www.guttmacher.org/fact-sheet
/state-facts-about-abortion-ohio#.

26. Phone interview with Michelle Davis, August 25, 2020.

27. Davis, interview.

28. Niraj Chokshi, "Ohio's Fetal Heartbeat Abortion Ban Is Latest
Front in Fight over Roe v. Wade," *The New York Times*, April
12, 2019, www.nytimes.com/2019/04/12/us/ohio-abortion
.html.

29. Jeff Zeleny, "Ohio's Republican Governor Intentionally Takes
Slow Approach as Other States Rush to Reopen," CNN,
May 1, 2020, www.cnn.com/2020/05/01/politics/ohio-mike
-dewine-may-reopen/index.html.

30. "RE: Director's Order for the Management of Non-Essential
Surgeries and Procedures Throughout Ohio," Ohio Department of Health, March 17, 2020, www.documentcloud.org
/documents/6816633-Director-s-Order-Non-Essential
-Surgery.html.

31. Kristina Sgueglia, Alta Spells, and Sheena Jones, "Ohio Orders Abortion Clinics to Stop 'Nonessential Abortions'

Because of Coronavirus," CNN, March 22, 2020, www.cnn
.com/2020/03/22/us/ohio-abortion-coronavirus/index.html.

32. Cornelius Frolik, "Coronavirus Crisis: Ohio Abortion Providers Say They Will Remain Open," *Dayton Daily News*, March 22,
2020, www.daytondailynews.com/news/local/coronavirus
-crisis-ohio-abortion-providers-say-they-will-remain-open
/spvJEOpG9zYTvQFM9WD8lJ.

33. Jarrod Clay, "Appeals Court Decision Will Allow Ohio Abortion Clinics to Remain Open During Pandemic," ABC6,
April 6, 2020, abc6onyourside.com/news/local/appeals-court
-decision-will-allow-ohio-abortion-clinics-to-remain-open
-during-pandemic.

34. Davis, interview.

35. Laurie Sobel, Amrutha Ramaswamy, Brittni Frederiksen,
and Alina Salganicoff, "State Action to Limit Abortion Access During the COVID-19 Pandemic," Kaiser Family Foundation, August 10, 2020, www.kff.org/coronavirus-covid-19
/issue-brief/state-action-to-limit-abortion-access-during-the
-covid-19-pandemic.

36. Phone interview with Bianca Cameron-Schwiesow, May 18,
2020.

37. Cameron-Schwiesow, interview.

38. "Radical Anti-Abortion Activists Descend on Alabama,"
Rolling Stone, July 28, 2015, www.rollingstone.com/politics
/politics-news/radical-anti-abortion-activists-descend-on
-alabama-61401.

39. Rebecca Grant, "How an Extremist Anti-Abortion Protest
Resulted in a Safe Haven for Women," *Vice*, October 24, 2016,
www.vice.com/en/article/7xzbyd/how-an-extremist-anti
-abortion-protest-resulted-in-a-safe-haven-for-women.

40. Associated Press Staff, "Abortion-Rape and Incest," *Observer-Reporter*, June 18, 2019, observer-reporter.com/abortion-rape-and-incest/image_0e13d660-91f8-11e9-b516-b3dc32ab7b4c.html.

41. Cameron-Schwiesow, interview.

42. Phone interview with Travis Jackson, September 2019.

43. Cameron-Schwiesow, interview.

44. Cameron-Schwiesow, interview.

45. Cameron-Schwiesow, interview.

46. "Famous Cases & Criminals: Eric Rudolph," FBI.gov, accessed September 22, 2020, www.fbi.gov/history/famous-cases/eric-rudolph.

47. "Full Text of Eric Rudolph's Confession," NPR, April 14, 2005.

48. "Eric Robert Rudolph Files Handwritten Appeal to Get Sentence Thrown Out," WSB-TV.com, June 25, 2020, www.wsbtv.com/news/local/eric-robert-rudolph-files-handwritten-appeal-get-sentence-thrown-out/464KNWMOOBBK3M2C77NK4ZS4II.

49. Marlene Lenthang, "Kyle Rittenhouse, Illinois Teen Who Allegedly Killed 2 Protesters, Makes 1st In-person Court Appearance," *ABC News*, March 21, 2021, abcnews.go.com/US/kyle-rittenhouse-illinois-teen-allegedly-killed-protesters-makes/story?id=77825979.

Chapter Six: A Sanctuary State of Mind

1. Rachel K. Jones, "As Danger to 'Roe' Grows, Many Voters May Not Even Know That Abortion Is Legal," Guttmacher Institute, September 20, 2018, www.guttmacher.org/article/2018/09/danger-roe-grows-many-voters-may-not-even-know-abortion-legal.

2. "State Facts About Abortion: New Jersey," Guttmacher

Institute, last updated January 2021, www.guttmacher.org /fact-sheet/state-facts-about-abortion-new-jersey.

3. Elizabeth Nash and Joerg Dreweke, "The U.S. Abortion Rate Continues to Drop: Once Again, State Abortion Restrictions Are Not the Main Driver," Guttmacher Institute, September 18, 2019, www.guttmacher.org/gpr/2019/09/us-abortion-rate -continues-drop-once-again-state-abortion-restrictions-are -not-main.

4. Melissa Goodman and Katharine Bodde, "New York City Clinic Access Law," New York Civil Liberties Union, February 28, 2011, www.nyclu.org/sites/default/files/Clinic%20 Access%20Memo.pdf.

5. Phone interview with Becca Ballenger, September 14, 2020.

6. Ballenger, interview.

7. Ballenger, interview.

8. Kirby Wilson, "Florida 'Disability Abortion' Bill Has Some Critics in the Disability Community," *Tampa Bay Times*, April 22, 2021, www.tampabay.com/news/florida-politics/2021/04 /22/florida-disability-abortion-bill-has-some-critics-in-the -disability-community.

9. Ballenger, interview.

10. "A.G. Schneiderman Files Lawsuit to End Persistent Harassment of Women Entering Women's Health Clinic in Queens," New York State Office of the Attorney General, June 20, 2017, ag.ny.gov/press-release/2017/ag-schneiderman-files-lawsuit -end-persistent-harassment-women-entering-womens.

11. Ballenger, interview.

12. Phone interview with Ashley Gray and "Jane Roe," September 16, 2020.

13. Robin Marty, "One City's 6 Month Quest to Take Its Sidewalks Back from Anti-Abortion Protesters," *ThinkProgress*, March

19, 2014, archive.thinkprogress.org/one-citys-6-month-quest -to-take-its-sidewalks-back-from-anti-abortion-protesters -ccdaa270cc84.

14. "Politics & Voting in Englewood, New Jersey," *BestPlaces .com*, accessed July 5, 2021, www.bestplaces.net/voting/city /new_jersey/englewood.

15. Emily Crockett, "New Jersey Town Passes Buffer Zone Af- ter Protesters Get Aggressive," *Rewire News Group*, March 19, 2014, rewire.news/article/2014/03/19/new-jersey-town-passes -buffer-zone-protesters-get-aggressive.

16. Crockett, "New Jersey Town Passes Buffer Zone After Pro- testers Get Aggressive."

17. Supreme Court of the United States, McCullen et al. v. Coakley, Attorney General of Massachusetts, et al., No. 12-1168, June 26, 2014, www.supremecourt.gov/opinions/13pdf/12-1168_6k47.pdf.

18. Gray, interview.

19. New York State Senate Bill S2796, Reproductive Health Act, www.nysenate.gov/legislation/bills/2017/S2796.

20. "Governor Cuomo Signs Legislation Protecting Women's Reproductive Rights," New York State Office of the Gover- nor, January 22, 2019, www.governor.ny.gov/news/governor -cuomo-signs-legislation-protecting-womens-reproductive -rights.

21. Bill Chappell, "Supreme Court Strikes Down Abortion Clinic 'Buffer Zone' Law," NPR, June 26, 2014, www.npr .org/sections/thetwo-way/2014/06/26/325806464/states -cant-mandate-buffer-zones-around-abortion-clinics-high -court-says.

22. Phone interview with Pearl Brady, September 10, 2020.

23. Ballenger, interview.

24. Jeffrey C. Mays, "Anti-Abortion Protesters at Queens Clinic Did Not Harass Patients, Judge Rules," *The New York Times*, July 22, 2018, www.nytimes.com/2018/07/22/nyregion/anti -abortion-protesters-queens-clinic.html.

25. Brady, interview.

26. Ballenger, interview.

27. Emily Crockett, "How One Lawmaker and One University Could Leave Missouri with Just One Abortion Clinic," *Vox,* November 21, 2015, www.vox.com/2015/11/20/9768592 /missouri-planned-parenthood.

28. "QuickFacts: Granite City, Illinois," United States Census, accessed September 29, 2020, www.census.gov/quickfacts /granitecitycityillinois.

29. Phone interview with Robin Frisella, September 24, 2020.

30. "Illinois Abortion Law Guide: What does the Reproductive Health Act Mean?" ABC-7 Chicago, June 14, 2019, abc7 chicago.com/illinois-abortion-law-in-laws/5345982.

31. "Presidential voting trends in Illinois," Ballotpedia, accessed October 22, 2020, ballotpedia.org/Presidential _voting_trends_in_Illinois.

32. "2016 Presidential Election Results," *The New York Times*, August 9, 2017, www.nytimes.com/elections/2016/results/president.

33. "Presidential Election Results: Biden Wins," *The New York Times*, November 3, 2020, www.nytimes.com/interactive/2020 /11/03/us/elections/results-president.html.

34. Angie Leventis Lourgos, "More than 5,500 Women Came to Illinois to Have an Abortion Last Year amid Growing Restrictions in the Midwest," *Chicago Tribune,* November 30, 2018, www .chicagotribune.com/news/ct-met-abortion-numbers-illinois -out-of-state-20181129-story.html.

35.   Phone interview with Amanda Ehrhardt, June 1, 2020.

36.   "Granite City, Illinois Population 2021," World Population Review, accessed September 24, 2020, worldpopulation review.com/us-cities/granite-city-il-population.

37.   Phone interview with Justine Colom, May 14, 2020.

38.   Phone interview with Alison Dreith, May 8, 2020.

39.   "Granite City, Illinois Population 2021," World Population Review.

40.   Phone interview with Mariceli Algeria, May 15, 2020.

41.   "St. Louis, MO Weather History: May 11, 2019," Weather Underground, www.wunderground.com/history/daily/KSTL/date/2019-5-11.

42.   Colom, interview.

43.   "QuickFacts: Chicago, Illinois," United States Census, accessed September 29, 2020, www.census.gov/quickfacts/fact/table/chicagocityillinois,US/PST045219.

44.   "2020 Election Results: Illinois," *Politico*, January 6, 2021, www.politico.com/2020-election/results/illinois.

45.   "Chicago, Illinois," AbortionFinder.org, accessed September 18, 2020, www.abortionfinder.org/results?location=chicago,%20il.

46.   "Fairview Heights Health Center of Fairview Heights, IL," Planned Parenthood, accessed September 19, 2020, www.planned parenthood.org/health-center/illinois/fairview-heights/62208/fairview-heights-health-center-2712-90770.

47.   United States Court of Appeals for the Seventh Circuit, Veronica Price, et al. v. City of Chicago.

48.   Phone interview with Jay Griffin, May 20, 2020.

49.   Griffin, interview.

50.   Ulisano, interview, April 24, 2020.

51.   Griffin, interview.

52. Griffin, interview.

53. Ulisano, interview, April 2019.

54. "About the Clinic Vest Project," Clinic Vest Project, accessed October 14, 2020, www.clinicvestproject.org/about-the-clinic-vest-project.html.

55. Ulisano, interview, April 24, 2020.

56. Text message to Lauren Rankin from Ashley Gray, August 20, 2019.

57. United States Court of Appeals for the Third Circuit, Jeryl Turco v. City of Englewood, New Jersey, No. 17-3716, August 19, 2019, www2.ca3.uscourts.gov/opinarch/173716p.pdf.

58. Phone interview with Christine Taylor, May 20, 2020.

Chapter Seven: A Clinic Escort Without a Country

1. Horn, interview.

2. Schoen, *Abortion After Roe*, 165.

3. Barb Berggoetz, "Post-abortion Backup Doctors Could Be Publicly Named Under Bill," *IndyStar*, January 29, 2014, www.indystar.com/story/news/2014/01/29/post-abortion-backup-doctors-could-be-publicly-named-under-bill/5036707.

4. Horn, interview.

5. Kevin Leininger, "Doctor Takes Hiatus from abortions in Fort Wayne," *South Bend Tribune*, December 27, 2013, www.southbendtribune.com/story/news/local/2013/12/27/doctor-takes-hiatus-from-abortions-in-fort-wayne/46599783.

6. Horn, interview.

7. "State Facts About Abortion: Indiana," Guttmacher Institute, accessed October 28, 2020, www.guttmacher.org/fact-sheet/state-facts-about-abortion-indiana.

8. Horn, interview.

9. Horn, interview.

10.   "About Choices Medical," Choices Medical Women's Center, accessed October 14, 2020, www.choicesmedical.com /about-us.

11.   "Communities Need Clinics 2020 Report," Abortion Care Network, abortioncarenetwork.org/wp-content/uploads/2020/12 /CommunitiesNeedClinics-2020.pdf.

12.   Supreme Court of the United States, Donald J. Trump, President of the United States, et al. v. International Refugee Assistance Project, et al., Donald J. Trump, President of the United States, et al. v. Hawaii, et al., No. 16-1436 and 16-1540, June 26, 2017, www.supremecourt.gov/opinions/16pdf/16-1436 _16hc.pdf.

13.   Amy Howe, "Anthony Kennedy, Swing Justice, Announces Retirement," *SCOTUSblog*, June 27, 2018, www.scotusblog .com/2018/06/anthony-kennedy-swing-justice-announces -retirement.

14.   Supreme Court of the United States, Obergefell et al. v Hodges, Director, Ohio Department of Health, et al., No. 14-556, June 26, 2015, www.supremecourt.gov/opinions /14pdf/14-556_3204.pdf.

15.   Brian Naylor, "Trump Backtracks on Comments About Abortion and 'Punishment' for Women," NPR, March 30, 2016, www.npr.org/2016/03/30/472444293/trump-calls-for -punishing-women-who-have-abortions-then-backtracks.

16.   Glenn Kessler, "Brett Kavanaugh and Allegations of Sexual Misconduct: The Complete List," *The Washington Post*, September 27, 2018, www.washingtonpost.com/politics/2018/09/27 /brett-kavanaugh-allegations-sexual-misconduct-complete-list.

17.   Julie Hirschfeld Davis, "Departure of Kennedy, 'Firewall for Abortion Rights,' Could End Roe v. Wade," *The New York*

Times, June 27, 2018, www.nytimes.com/2018/06/27/us
/politics/kennedy-abortion-roe-v-wade.html.

18. Lauren Rankin, "Republican Leaders Asked the Supreme
Court to End Legal Abortion. They May Get Their Wish,"
NBC News, January 3, 2020, www.nbcnews.com/think
/opinion/republican-leaders-asked-supreme-court-end-legal
-abortion-they-may-ncna1110146.

19. Supreme Court of the United States, June Medical Services
L.L.C. et al. v. Russo, Interim Secretary, Louisiana Department of Health and Hospitals, No. 18-1323, June 29, 2020,
www.supremecourt.gov/opinions/19pdf/18-1323_c07d.pdf.

20. Phone interview with Ali Taylor, November 3, 2020.

21. Andrew DeMillo, "Court Lifts Block on 4 Arkansas Abortion Restrictions," Associated Press, August 7, 2020, apnews
.com/article/reproductive-rights-health-ar-state-wire-u-s
-supreme-court-arkansas-35d85111a05fcaf86ff2b0fa791136af.

22. Ali Taylor, interview.

23. Gabriella Borter, "Arkansas Passes Ban on All Abortions
Except in Medical Emergencies," Reuters, March 9, 2021,
www.reuters.com/business/healthcare-pharmaceuticals
/arkansas-passes-ban-all-abortions-except-medical-emergencies
-2021-03-09.

24. Supreme Court of the United States, Shelby County, Alabama
v. Holder, Attorney General, et al., No. 12-96, June 25, 2013,
www.supremecourt.gov/opinions/12pdf/12-96_6k47.pdf.

25. Nina Totenberg, "Justice Ruth Bader Ginsburg, Champion
of Gender Equality, Dies at 87," NPR, September 18, 2020,
www.npr.org/2020/09/18/100306972/justice-ruth-bader
-ginsburg-champion-of-gender-equality-dies-at-87.

26. Phone interview with Valerie Peterson, May 19, 2020.

27. Texas House Bill 2, July 18, 2013, capitol.texas.gov/tlo docs/832/billtext/html/HB00002F.HTM.

28. Valerie Peterson, "How Did I Get an Abortion in Texas? I Didn't," *The New York Times*, June 15, 2016, www.nytimes .com/2016/06/15/opinion/how-did-i-get-an-abortion-in -texas-i-didnt.html.

29. "Gretchen Dyer," IMDB, accessed November 1, 2020, www .imdb.com/name/nm0245726.

30. WFAA Staff, "Gretchen Dyer: Her Work Lifted Independent Filmmaking in N. Texas," WFAA.com, October 16, 2009, www.wfaa.com/article/news/local/gretchen-dyer-her-work -lifted-independent-filmmaking-in-n-texas/411394042.

31. Phone interview with Steve Leary, May 7, 2020.

32. Phone interview with Alyssa "Roscoe," May 13, 2020.

33. "Roscoe," interview.

34. "Roscoe," interview.

35. Leary, interview.

36. Phone interview with Steph Black, October 6, 2020.

37. DMV Abortion Practical Support Network, dapsn.wordpress .com.

38. Black, interview.

39. Black, interview.

40. "State Bans on Abortion Throughout Pregnancy," Guttmacher Institute, last updated June 1, 2021, www.guttmacher .org/state-policy/explore/state-policies-later-abortions.

41. "Induced Abortion in the United States, September 2019 Fact Sheet," Guttmacher Institute, accessed August 28, 2020, www .guttmacher.org/fact-sheet/induced-abortion-united-states.

42. *People* Staff, "I Thought Abortion Restrictions Were a Reasonable Compromise—Until I Needed One at 32," *People*, March

4, 2020, people.com/health/i-thought-abortion-restrictions
-were-a-reasonable-compromise-until-i-needed-one-at-32
-weeks.

43. *People* Staff, "I Thought Abortion Restrictions Were a Reasonable Compromise."

44. Phone interview with Odile Schalit, October 30, 2020.

45. "About Access Reproductive Justice," ACCESS Reproductive Justice, accessrj.org/about-access-reproductive-justice/.

46. Schalit, interview.

47. "How Hyde Hurts Women," *Conscience Magazine*, Issue 2, December 3, 2015, www.catholicsforchoice.org/resource -library/how-hyde-hurts-women.

48. Phone interview with Renee Bracey Sherman, March 26, 2019.

Chapter Eight: How Do You Solve a Problem Like Abortion?

1. Jeanne Clark, interview.

2. Jeanne Clark, interview.

3. Lisa Greenhouse, "Court Rules Abortion Clinics Can Use Rackets Law to Sue," *The New York Times*, January 25, 1994, www .nytimes.com/1994/01/25/us/court-rules-abortion-clinics -can-use-rackets-law-to-sue.html.

4. Linda Greenhouse, "Supreme Court Voids Racketeering Conviction of Anti-Abortion Groups in 80's Case," *The New York Times*, February 27, 2003, www.nytimes.com/2003/02/27 /us/supreme-court-voids-racketeering-conviction-of-anti -abortion-groups-in-80-s-case.html.

5. "Justice Amy Coney Barrett Swearing-In Ceremony at the White House," C-SPAN, October 26, 2020, www.c-span .org/video/?477418-1/justice-amy-coney-barrett-sworn -justice-clarence-thomas.

6.   Barbara Sprunt, "Amy Coney Barrett Confirmed to Su-
      preme Court, Takes Constitutional Oath," NPR, October 26,
      2020, www.npr.org/2020/10/26/927640619/senate-confirms
      -amy-coney-barrett-to-the-supreme-court.

7.   Josh Salman and Kevin McCoy, "Supreme Court Nominee
      Amy Barrett Signed Anti-abortion Letter Accompanying
      Ad Calling to Overturn Roe v. Wade," *USA Today*, Octo-
      ber 1, 2020, www.usatoday.com/story/news/2020/10/01/amy
      -barrett-signed-anti-abortion-letter-alongside-anti-roe-v
      -wade-ad/5880595002.

8.   Elizabeth Nash and Lauren Cross, "2021 Is on Track to Be-
      come the Most Devastating Antiabortion State Legislative
      Session in Decades," Guttmacher Institute, April 2021, www
      .guttmacher.org/article/2021/04/2021-track-become-most
      -devastating-antiabortion-state-legislative-session-decades.

9.   Rachel K. Jones and Jenna Jerman, "Abortion Incidence and
      Service Availability in the United States, 2014," *Perspectives on
      Sexual and Reproductive Health*, Vol. 49, Issue 1, March 2017,
      doi/full/10.1363/psrh.12015.

10.   Elizabeth Nash, "State Abortion Policy Landscape: From
      Hostile to Supportive," Guttmacher Institute, August 2019,
      www.guttmacher.org/article/2019/08/state-abortion-policy
      -landscape-hostile-supportive.

11.   Phone interview with Erin Matson, June 22, 2020.

12.   Kate Sheppard, "The Abortion Wars Come to Mary-
      land," *Mother Jones*, August 3, 2011, www.motherjones.com
      /politics/2011/08/leroy-carhart-summer-of-mercy.

13.   Sarah Kliff, "Why LeRoy Carhart Won't Stop Doing Abor-
      tions," *Newsweek*, August 14, 2009, www.newsweek.com
      /why-leroy-carhart-wont-stop-doing-abortions-79037.

14. Carrie Johnson, "Justice Department Tougher on Abortion Protesters," NPR, September 1, 2011, www.npr.org/2011/09 /01/140094051/obama-takes-tougher-stance-on-abortion -protesters.

15. Kliff, "Why LeRoy Carhart Won't Stop Doing Abortions."

16. Dan Harris, Huma Khan, Ariane de Vogue, "Nebraska Passes Controversial Abortion Ban," *ABC News*, April 13, 2010, abcnews.go.com/WN/Supreme_Court/nebraska-passes -controversial-abortion-ban/story?id=10361705.

17. Ed Pilkington, "I Shot US Abortion Doctor to Protect Children, Scott Roeder tells court," *The Guardian*, January 28, 2010, www .theguardian.com/world/2010/jan/28/scott-roeder-abortion -doctor-killer.

18. Matson, interview.

19. Matson, interview.

20. Matson, interview.

21. Supreme Court of the United States, Planned Parenthood of Southeastern Pennsylvania v. Casey, No. 91-744, June 29, 1992, www.oyez.org/cases/1991/91-744.

22. Supreme Court of the United States, Gonzales v. Carhart, No. 05-380, November 8, 2006, www.oyez.org/cases/2006 /05-380.

23. "U.S. Public Continues to Favor Legal Abortion, Oppose Overturning Roe v. Wade," Pew Research Center, August 29, 2019, www.pewresearch.org/politics/2019/08/29/u-s-public -continues-to-favor-legal-abortion-oppose-overturning-roe -v-wade.

24. Supreme Court of the United States, Planned Parenthood of Southeastern Pennsylvania v. Casey.

25. Elizabeth Nash, Rachel Benson Gold, Lizamarie Mohammed,

Zohra Ansari-Thomas, Olivia Cappello, "Policy Trends in the States, 2017," Guttmacher Institute, January 2018, www .guttmacher.org/article/2018/01/policy-trends-states-2017.

26. Maggie Astor, "What Is the Hyde Amendment? Look at Its Impact as Biden Reverses His Stance," *The New York Times*, June 7, 2019, www.nytimes.com/2019/06/07/us/politics /what-is-the-hyde-amendment.html.

27. "Communities Need Clinics 2020 Report," Abortion Care Network, 9-10, abortioncarenetwork.org/wp-content/uploads /2020/12/CommunitiesNeedClinics-2020.pdf.

28. "Medication Abortion," Guttmacher Institute, last updated June 1, 2021, www.guttmacher.org/state-policy/explore /medication-abortion.

29. "Self-Managed Abortion and the Law," Repro Legal Help-line, accessed November 16, 2020, www.reprolegalhelpline .org/self-managed-abortion-and-the-law.

30. "How to Get Abortion Pills," Plan C Pills, accessed September 30, 2020, www.plancpills.org/guide-how-to-get-abortion -pills.

31. Black, interview.

32. Aid Access website, aidaccess.org/en/i-need-an-abortion.

33. Abigail R. A. Aiken, Jennifer E. Starling, Rebecca Gomperts, Mauricio Tec, James G. Scott, Catherine E. Aiken, "De-mand for Self-Managed Online Telemedicine Abortion in the United States During the Coronavirus Disease 2019 (COVID-19) Pandemic," *Obstetrics and Gynecology*, Vol. 136, Issue 4, October 2020, 835–837, journals.lww.com/green journal/Fulltext/2020/10000/Demand_for_Self_Managed_ Online_Telemedicine.29.aspx.

34. Amy Gastelum, "Purvi Patel Faces 20 Years in Prison for

Feticide and Child Neglect," *The World*, March 31, 2015, www.pri.org/node/78896/popout.

35. Susan Rinkunas, "Indiana Court Throws Out Purvi Patel's Abortion Conviction, *The Cut*, July 22, 2016, www.thecut .com/2016/07/court-throws-out-purvi-patel-feticide-conviction .html.

36. Lauren Rankin, "How an Online Search for Abortion Pills Landed This Woman in Jail," *Fast Company*, February 26, 2020, www.fastcompany.com/90468030/how-an-online-search-for -abortion-pills-landed-this-woman-in-jail.

37. Matson, interview.

38. Ulisano, interview, April 2019.

39. Matson, interview.

40. Hagstrom Miller, interview, May 18, 2020.

41. Phone interview with Liz Gustafson, May 12, 2020.

42. "Induced Abortion in the United States Fact Sheet: September 2019," Guttmacher Institute, www.guttmacher.org/fact-sheet /induced-abortion-united-states.

43. K. M. Shellenberg, *Abortion Stigma in the United States: Quantitative and Qualitative Perspectives from Women Seeking an Abortion* (Baltimore, MD: Johns Hopkins University, 2010).

44. Corinne H. Rocca, Goleen Samari, Diana G. Foster, Heather Gould, Katrina Kimport, "Emotions and Decision Rightness over Five Years Following an Abortion: An Examination of Decision Difficulty and Abortion Stigma," *Social Science & Medicine*, Vol. 248, March 2020, doi.org/10.1016/j .socscimed.2019.112704.

45. Gustafson, interview.

46. Gretchen Sisson and Katrina Kimport, "Telling Stories About Abortion: Abortion-Related Plots in American Film and

Television 1916–2013," *Contraception*, 89(5): 413-8, May 2014, pubmed.ncbi.nlm.nih.gov/24512938.

47.   Suzanne Zane et al., "Abortion-Related Mortality in the United States 1998–2010," *Obstetrics & Gynecology*, Vol. 126, Issue 2, August 2015, 258–265, www.ncbi.nlm.nih.gov/pmc /articles/PMC4554338.

48.   "Abortion Onscreen Report 2019," Advancing New Standards in Reproductive Health (ANSIRH), www.ansirh.org/sites /default/files/publications/files/Abortion%20Onscreen%20 Report%202019.pdf.

49.   Ariana Romero, "Why Aidy Bryant's Hulu Comedy *Shrill* Took Just 20 Minutes to Show An Abortion," *Refinery29*, March 15, 2019, www.refinery29.com/en-us/2019/03/226974 /shrill-hulu-season-1-premiere-recap-annie-abortion-ryan-baby.

50.   Sesali Bowen, "*Broad City* Perfectly Captured the Climate for Young Women Post-Election," *Refinery29*, September 21, 2017, www.refinery29.com/en-us/2017/09/173252 /broad-city-season-4-episode-2-abortion-clinic.

51.   Lauren Rankin, "What 'Black Mirror' Got So Wrong About Emergency Contraception and Abortion," *SELF*, January 3, 2018, www.self.com/story/what-black-mirror-gets-so-wrong -about-emergency-contraception-and-abortion.

52.   Renee Bracey Sherman, "One in Four Women Have Abortions. Why Don't We Talk About It?" *BillMoyers.com*, November 12, 2017, billmoyers.com/story/creating-common -ground-abortion-stories-love-compassion.

53.   Horowitz, interview.

54.   Phone interview with Paula Harris, May 11, 2020.

55.   Barrett, interview, April 21, 2020.

56.   Barrett, interview, April 21, 2020.

57.   Barrett, interview, April 21, 2020.

EPILOGUE: Hindsight Is 2020

1.   APM Research Lab Staff, "The Color of Coronavirus: COVID-19 Deaths by Race and Ethnicity in the U.S.," March 5, 2021, www.apmresearchlab.org/covid/deaths-by-race.

2.   Associated Press Staff. "Doctor Is No Stranger to Physical Threats: A Pipe Bomb Severely Damaged His Clinic in 1986. His Sign Outside the Rubble Read, 'Hell, No. We Won't Go!' He's Been Frequent Target of Protests," *Los Angeles Times*, August 21, 1993, www.latimes.com/archives/la-xpm-1993-08-21-mn-26045-story.html.

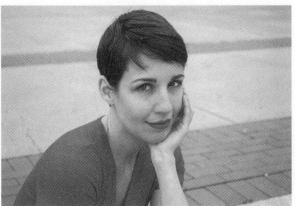

LAUREN RANKIN is a writer, speaker, and expert on abortion rights in the United States. Her work has been featured in *The Washington Post*, *TIME*, *The Cut*, *Fast Company*, *Teen Vogue*, *Refinery29*, *NBC News*, and many other publications. She spent six years as an abortion clinic escort in northern New Jersey, and is a board member of A is For, a reproductive rights advocacy organization. She lives in Longmont, Colorado, with her family. Find out more at laurenarankin.com.